3D Automated Breast Volume Sonography

Veronika Gazhonova

3D Automated Breast Volume Sonography

A Practical Guide

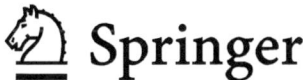 Springer

Veronika Gazhonova
Department of Radiology Chair
Central State Medical Academy
Department of Radiology
Moscow
Russia

The Work was first published in 2015 by the author with the following title:
Ультразвуковой томосинтез молочных желез

ISBN 978-3-319-41970-1   ISBN 978-3-319-41971-8   (eBook)
DOI 10.1007/978-3-319-41971-8

Library of Congress Control Number: 2016959475

Printed on acid-free paper

This Springer imprint is published by Springer Nature
The registered company is Springer International Publishing AG Switzerland
The registered company address is Gewerbestrasse 11, 6330 Cham, Switzerland

To my husband Alexander and daughters Olga and Julia in gratitude for their patience and support.

Foreword I

Rapid scientific and technological advances have fundamentally changed the face of modern medicine. This applies completely to breast visualization technologies. New opportunities have been opened up by digital technology. Currently, the arsenal of breast diagnostic visualization contains not only the traditional X-ray (mammography) and ultrasound techniques but also X-ray-free beam methods, Doppler sonography, automated breast volume sonography (ABVS) tomography, multispiral CT, MR tomography, as well as hybrid techniques.

However, despite the wide range of visualization methods available to the modern physician at present, clinical breast health medicine does not have a universal way to retrieve medical information that provides answers to all the questions of a radiologist in a breast examination. Of special interest is the presurgical differential diagnosis of clinically occult and non-palpable early forms of benign and malignant breast diseases.

This publication reflects the latest achievements in the field of ultrasound diagnostic technology, that is, ultrasound tomosynthesis. The author summarizes the materials of her own research and presents the best technological and methodical practices for obtaining breast structure images and features of their interpretation in view of the new possibilities in reconstruction of sectional images. The symptom complexes characteristic for different diseases are described, as are errors due to technical biases or incorrect interpretation of the information obtained. The extensive illustrative material clearly shows the potential of the new technology.

This publication will provide valuable knowledge for doctors of different specialties: oncomammologists, obstetricians-gynecologists, oncologists, general practitioners, and ultrasound diagnosticians.

I wish you success on the path of learning and training!

The head of the National Center for Oncology of Reproductive Organs of the Moscow Research Oncological Institute named after PA Herzen (MNIOI), branch of "NMIRC" of the Ministry of Health of Russia, honored scientific worker of the RF, USSR Council of Ministers award winner, president of the Russian Association of Oncology, president of the Russian Association of Radiologists, and doctor of medical sciences, Professor N.I. Rozhkova

> From the birth of a child to the later years of life the breast repeatedly changes its appearance: starting with a small bud, it passes through an exhilarating flourishing, and concludes its time in withered tranquility. The X-ray image of the breast of every woman is unique. Prof. LD. Lindenbraten
>
> People only see what they are prepared to see. Ralph Jefferson

3D automated whole breast sonography is a rather new method that was approved for clinical studies in 2009. The idea of covering the whole organ in one ultrasound scan is unique for the breast, and automation helps in overcoming two inherent limitations of ultrasound: small field of view and poor reproducibility. The new 3D ultrasound technique is still at the stage of investigation regarding its effectiveness in screening programs, and this book will be very helpful in providing knowledge for less experienced and new users of 3D ABVS, thus contributing to its wider clinical integration. With this in mind, much attention was paid in this book to technical aspects, patient positioning, image analysis, and comparison of this new technique with standard handheld ultrasound and mammography.

This book introduces an exciting new method of diagnostic breast ultrasound – automated whole-breast volume scanning (3D ABVS). It is the first practical guide dedicated to the use of this new technique. I believe that this book will assist in learning it and provide guidance to users of 3D ABVS in the clinical setting.

I was impressed by the convincing demonstration of the advantages of the new method for diagnosis of breast cancer in women with dense glandular tissue. Comparisons of 3D ABVS images with findings on X-ray mammography and conventional 2D handheld US are impressive and aid in understanding the benefits of the method.

This book summarizes the accumulated knowledge on ABVS but stands apart from other publications on this topic. The author recommends modifying patient positioning and the acquisition technique in order to make 3D ABVS images comparable to standard mammographic projections.

Bernd Hamm, MD
Professor and Chair
Departments of Radiology
Campus Charité Mitte/Campus Virchow-Klinikum/
Campus Benjamin Franklin
Charité – Universitätsmedizin Berlin
Humboldt-Universität zu Berlin and Freie Universität Berlin
Berlin, Germany

Preface

Frequent advances in transducer design, electronics, computers, and signal processing have improved the quality of ultrasound images to the extent that sonography is now a major mode of imaging for clinical diagnosis of breast cancer. New opportunities for automation in combination with three-dimensional reconstruction have opened up a new era in breast ultrasound. This new technique is called automated breast volume sonography (ABVS) or "breast sono-tomosynthesis."

In order to understand how it works, one should sum up and assess its capabilities. From a practical point of view, sono-tomosynthesis is very close to digital X-ray breast tomosynthesis. The introduction of this technology into clinical practice will require additional training of not only US specialists but also radiologists. Anticipating a new phase in diagnostic breast imaging, we attempted to analyze the available knowledge and develop practical guidance on ABVS tomography. This book will be helpful not only for ABVS beginners but also for advanced ABVS users. A detailed description is provided of ABVS tomography indications, scanning technique, patient positioning, protocols, image analysis, X-ray comparisons, and normal breast anatomy with ABVS. Also we provide clinical examples of ABVS in benign and malignant tumors, in inflammatory processes, in postoperative breast changes, and in breast augmentation. Limitations of the method are also described and illustrated. The book is illustrated by the author's own clinical observations and interesting cases provided courtesy of specialists wishing to share their findings, to whom the author expresses her cordial thanks.

We hope that this book will be useful not only for US diagnostics specialists and radiologists but also for physicians involved in the diagnostic algorithm of evaluation and treatment of breast disease.

Moscow, Russia   Veronika Gazhonova, MD PhD

Acknowledgement

The author thanks for the help with images:

Group of authors: Rozhkova NI, Mazo ML, and Yakobs OE (from the National Center for Oncology of Reproductive Organs of the Moscow Research Oncological Institute named after PA Herzen (MNIOI), branch of "NMIRC" of the Ministry of Health of Russia) with pictures to Chap. 4 (Fig. 4.50) and (Fig. 4.60)

Vasilchenko SA (from the Federal State Budget Organization "Polyclinic №3" under the General Management Department of the president of the Russian Federation) to Chap. 4 (Fig. 4.54) and (Fig. 4.56)

The author cordially thanks for the pictures that were provided by those researchers.

Introduction

Breast cancer is the most frequent malignant tumor in women, diagnosed in approximately 1.4 million people each year with a steadily growing incidence [1]. The number of newly diagnosed breast cancer cases is increasing yearly. In the structure of women's cancer mortality, breast cancer occupies the leading positions [1, 2]. The survival rate is known to be directly dependent on the proper cancer treatment and on the stage of the disease. The overall survival of adequately treated patients with noninvasive breast cancer approaches 100%, while the 5-year survival of patients with stage IV breast cancer is less than 10% [3]. This implies the need to develop noninvasive diagnostic methods for qualifying non-palpable breast masses, and that is still a priority of modern mammology. Manifestations of breast cancer are so diverse that only comprehensive examination with X-ray mammography (MMG) at the first stage followed by ultrasound (US) allows the detection of specific signs indicating breast malignancy.

X-ray mammography is currently the "gold standard" for breast cancer screening due to being a quick, inexpensive, easily reproducible, objective, and operator-independent method allowing detection of preclinical breast cancer with the most favorable prognosis [4]. However, the diagnostic possibilities of X-ray mammography in breast cancer detection decrease in relation to breast density. In the case of dense breast tissue, the sensitivity of X-ray MMG reduces by up to 48% [5].

Handheld US (HHUS) is widely available for breast studies and well tolerated due to modern sensitive high-frequency transducers, improvement of Doppler technology and elastography, and development of ABVS tomography. A large multicenter trial has demonstrated that screening with HHUS finds significantly more early-stage breast cancers than screening with mammography alone and has a cancer detection rate of 0.3–0.5% [6–8]. However, handheld breast US is known to be time-consuming and lacking standardized techniques, operator dependent, and poorly reproducible [9].

ABUS is an option proposed to overcome the time-consuming and costly nature of handheld, physician-performed whole-breast US (WBUS). Innovative technologies for automatic breast scanning ensure consistently high-quality images covering the entire breast from the top of the nipple to the chest wall using three-dimensional techniques. Automation reduces the duration of the study. This will present a considerable advantage and savings potential, especially for screening programs.

Interest in evaluation of the possibilities of ABVS is growing worldwide. However, there has been limited research on the applicability of ABUS because of the differences in the technique, data acquisition, and interpretation [10]. Automated breast US (ABUS) was introduced more than a decade ago; at that time, the image quality of the scans was not sufficiently good to interpret the results. However, 5 years later, modern ABUS scanners using high-frequency transducers were introduced and have improved image quality. Over the 5-year experience of the technique, less than 40 papers have been published concerning ABVS performance. High reproducibility and high sensitivity of the method in breast cancer detection were reported [11–20]. In September 2012, the US Food and Drug Administration (US FDA) approved an ABUS system (somo-v ABUS, U-Systems) to be used for whole-breast US screening after negative findings using mammography in women with dense breasts who had not previously undergone surgery or biopsy [21]. Recent breast density legislation in the USA has continued to increase the demand for supplemental US screening [22].

The studies of American scientists showed that combined use of two methods—X-ray mammography and 3D US—allowed the detection of more cancers in women with breast cancer risk factors and dense glandular tissue. The inclusion of 3D US in screening additionally improved the sensitivity of detection of tumors up to 77.5 % [23].

This high sensitivity of ABVS is enabled by identifying the "retraction" phenomenon in a coronal slice. This symptom, according to Lin X et al., has 100 % specificity, 80 % sensitivity, and 91.4 % accuracy in differentiating benign and malignant masses [14]. However, before the era of 3D breast ultrasound, it was not possible to see this phenomenon using conventional 2D ultrasound. Various mechanical artifacts arising while collecting 3D US data precluded the complete identification and assessment of the significance of the findings in the US diagnosis of breast cancer. The initial experience of clinical studies of ABVS in Russia has also shown encouraging results: no cases of breast cancer were missed [17, 18–20]. ABVS showed 100 % sensitivity, 40 % specificity, and 88 % accuracy of detection of breast pathology. Further clinical studies are needed to evaluate the performance of the automated breast scanning system [17, 20].

The advantages of the automatic breast scanning process include standardization with the possibility of second look and follow-up studies, reproducibility, and operator independence. The quality of ABVS images produced in standard projections is independent of the operator. 3D information can be acquired by any trained person, regardless of the level of training, whereas the usual study should be performed by a qualified physician or sonographer with knowledge of the basics of ultrasound and anatomy of the breast. Automation reduces the duration of each study to an average of 15 min, which is less than that of a conventional breast study. This allows proper organization of patient flow in outpatient departments and reduces waiting time by increasing the capacity of radiology departments. With sufficient experience in the interpretation of 3D images, an experienced doctor will be able to document a simple case in 10 min and a more complicated one in about 20 min.

An automated wide aperture transducer fully covers the entire breast and provides a global view of the breast anatomy, includes a large mass in one scan, or adequately depicts multifocal and multicentric cancer. The method performs measurements more accurately, which is important for follow-up studies, such as in the cases of neoadjuvant chemotherapy. Coronal slices of the breast obtained from the tip of the nipple to the chest wall are unique, allowing quick identification of areas with impaired architecture in a single image.

We have developed a standardized algorithm for using ABVS for the diagnosis of breast cancer by comparing ABVS data with X-ray mammography. We have proposed a unified scanning standard and suggested special positions to obtain better ABVS tomograms, which allow the comparison of 3D ABVS tomogram slices with the standard projections in X-ray MMG. We also suggested possible indications and evaluated typical disadvantages and advantages of the new method in the diagnosis of cancer and various breast diseases.

Literature

1. Čissov VI, Starinskij VV, Petrova GV (2012) Malignant neoplasm in Russia in 2012 (morbidity and mortality). P. Moscow Oncology Research Institute named by NA Herzen, Moscow (book in Russian)
2. Malignant neoplasm in Russia (morbidity and mortality): the statistical compendium (2012) Ministry of Health of the Russian Federation/ed. by the Akad of RAMS Chissov VI et al.—Moscow: Center for informational technology and epidemiological studies in the field of oncology (book in Russian)
3. Axel EM (2006) Malignant neoplasm of the breast: the state of cancer care, morbidity, and mortality. Mammology 1:9–13 (article in Russian)
4. Rozhkova NI (ed) (2013) X-ray diagnosis in mammology: guide for physicians. SIMK, Moscow (article in Russian)
5. Duijm LE, Louwman MW, Groenewoud JH et al (2009) Inter-observer variability in mammography screening and effect of type and number of readers on screening outcome. Br J Cancer 13(6):901–907
6. Berg WA, Blume JD, Cormack JB et al (2008) Combined screening with ultrasound and mammography vs mammography alone in women at elevated risk of breast cancer. JAMA 299:2151–2163
7. Buchberger W, Niehoff A, Obrist P et al (2000) Clinically and mammographically occult breast lesions: detection and classification with high resolution sonography. Semin Ultrasound CT MR 21:325–336
8. Kolb TM, Lichy J, Newhouse JH (2002) Comparison of the performance of screening mammography, physical examination, and breast US and evaluation of factors that influence them: an analysis of 27,825 patient evaluations. Radiology 225:165–175
9. Berg WA, Blume JD, Cormack JB, Mendelson EB (2006) Operator dependence of physician-performed whole-breast US: lesion detection and characterization. Radiology 241:355–365
10. Shin HJ (2015) Current status of automated breast ultrasonography. Ultrasonography 34(3):165–172. http://dx.doi.org/10.14366/usg.15002
11. Kelly KM, Dean J, Lee SJ et al (2010) Breast cancer detection: radiologists' performance using mammography with and without automated whole-breast ultrasound. Eur Radiol 20:2557–2564
12. Shin HJ, Kim HH, Cha JH et al (2011) Automated ultrasound of the breast for diagnosis: interobserver agreement on lesion detection and characterization. AJR Am J Roentgenol 197:747–754
13. Wojcinski S, Farrokh A, Hille U et al (2011) The automated breast volume scanner (ABVS): initial experiences in lesion detection compared with conventional handheld B-mode ultrasound: a pilot study of 50 cases. Int J Women's Health 13:337–346

14. Lin X, Wang J, Han F et al (2012) Analysis of eighty-one cases with breast lesions using automated breast volume scanner and comparison with handheld ultrasound. Eur J Radiol 13(5):873–878

15. Wojcinski S, Gyapong S, Farrokh A et al (2013) Diagnostic performance and inter-observer concordance in lesion detection with the automated breast volume scanner (ABVS). BMC Med Imaging 13:36

16. Golatta M, Franz D, Harcos A et al (2013) Interobserver reliability of automated breast volume scanner (ABVS) interpretation and agreement of ABVS findings with hand held breast ultrasound (HHUS), mammography and pathology results. Eur J Radiol 13(8):332–336

17. Jacobs OE, Rozhkova NI, Maso ML et al (2014) An experience of virtual sonography of the breast use. Ann Roentgenol Radiol 1:23–32 (article in Russian)

18. Gazhonova VE, Bachurina EM, Khlustina EM et al (2014) Automatic sonotomography of mammary glands (3D ABVS). Part 1. Integration of US method in the radiological imaging standards. Polyclinic Radiol 3:342–348 (article in Russian)

19. Golatta M, Baggs C, Schweitzer-Martin M et al (2015) Evaluation of an automated breast 3D-ultrasound system by comparing it with hand-held ultrasound (HHUS) and mammography. Arch Gynecol Obstet 291:889–895

20. Gazhonova VE, Efremova MP, Khlustina EM (2015) Automatic sonotomography of mammary glands (Automated Volume Breast Sonography) – a new method of cancer diagnostics. Medical Visualization 2:67–77 (article in Russian)

21. U.S. Food and Drug Administration. Medical devices: somo-v Automated Breast Ultrasound System (ABUS): P110006 [Internet]. Silver Spring, MD: U.S. Food and Drug Administration. 2012. [cited 2014 Apr 10]. Available from: http://www.fda.gov/MedicalDevices/ProductsandMedicalProcedures/DeviceApprovalsandClearances/Recently-ApprovedDevices/ucm320724.htm.]

22. Skaane P, Gullien R, Eben EB et al (2015) Interpretation of automated breast ultrasound (ABUS) with and without knowledge of mammography: a reader performance study. Acta Radiol 56:404–412

23. ACR practice guideline for the performance of a breast ultrasound examination (2011) American College of Radiology. Revised 2011 (Resolution 11) [Internet] Reston, VA: American College of Radiology

Abbreviations

ABVS	Automated breast volume sonography
AP	Anteroposterior view (corresponds to ABVS)
Axilla	Axillaris oblique view (corresponds to ABVS)
BC	Breast cancer
CC	Craniocaudal (corresponds to mammogram)
CT	Computed tomography
DBT	Digital breast tomosynthesis
DCIS	Ductal carcinoma in situ
HHUS	Handheld ultrasound
IDC	Invasive ductal carcinoma
Inf	Inferior-to-superior view (corresponds to ABVS)
L AP	Left anteroposterior view (corresponds to ABVS)
Lat	Latero-medial oblique view (corresponds to ABVS)
LCIS	Lobular carcinoma in situ
Med	Mediolateral oblique view (corresponds to ABVS)
MLo	Mediolateral oblique (corresponds to mammogram)
MMG	Mammography
MRI	Magnetic resonance tomography
R AP	Right anteroposterior view (corresponds to ABVS)
Sup	Superior-to-inferior view (corresponds to ABVS)
TN	Triple negative
US	Ultrasound

Contents

The concept of automated breast US dates back to the 1970s when the first usable systems were reported by Maturo et al. [1]. All automatic US breast scanners have been classified as prone-type or supine-type scanners [2]. The first method used a special water bath-type scanning, the second carried out water-coupled scanning. Old generation automated scanners were of inferior quality with relatively low-frequency transducers of 4–7 MHz [3].

Interest in obtaining three-dimensional images of the breast has increased since the early 1990s after the development of powerful computer programs. Currently 3D imaging is a daily routine all over the world.

At the moment the possibility of computer-aided breast studies is provided by several US diagnostic systems, most of which unfortunately are not certified in the Russian market, although actively and widely used throughout the world, having Food and Drug Administration (FDA) approval. Comparative characteristics of these diagnostic systems are summarized in Table 1.1.

The first hybrid system included a 2D high-resolution sensor, mounted on a special stand to perform automatic scans [4]. This device was not equipped with a special wide aperture transducer, and scanning was performed mechanically, by moving the conventional transducer over the breast, in a way similar to that used for handheld ultrasound (HHUS). A special silicone pad was applied to facilitate sliding on the breast. This system was approved by the FDA in 2008 for clinical use in the USA [5]. The robotic device could convert from 2000 to 5000 2D axial scans into a 3D image. The first fundamental scientific works and mass screenings using automatic 3D scans were performed on this hybrid system. Several studies using such an ABUS system have been published, showing no improvement in detection of breast cancer in screening programs [6–8]. The disadvantages of the method included the impossibility of subsequent reconstructions of 3D images obtained and the inability to restore the initially collected 2D data from the combined array. The image was analyzed in real time, similar to any standard US examination.

An example of modern equipment for automatic 3D scanning is the Acuson S2000 automated breast volume scanner (ABVS) system from Siemens AG. The American company U-Systems, Inc., a manufacturer of ultrasound equipment for breast examinations, has developed a special transducer for breast examinations (automated breast ultrasound, abbr. ABUS). In Europe, Siemens AG has developed its Acuson S2000 ABVS system, based on U-Systems technology, and it is the first commercial product of its type on the Russian market (Fig. 1.1).

This scanner uses a completely different principle to obtain automated breast images than the previous hybrid system. It is equipped with a special high-frequency and wide-field-of-view, large footprint (15×17 cm) transducer attached to the US unit as a separate stand-alone device. This transducer is similar in size and shape to a

© Springer International Publishing Switzerland 2017
V. Gazhonova, *3D Automated Breast Volume Sonography*, DOI 10.1007/978-3-319-41971-8_1

Table 1.1 Comparison of US devices for automatic breast scanning

Type of device	SonoCine (hybrid)	Invenia ABUS (GE), ACUSON S2000 ABVS (Siemens)	Combined US system (Ultrasonix)
Scanning type	Conventional US sensor mounted on a handle	Large transducer with a special compression paddle	Concave sensor built into a couch, rotating 360°
Patient position during the study	Supine	Supine	Prone
With which radiological technique it could be integrated	N/A	Possible with MMG at compatible scans	CT, MRI
Acquisition time	15–30 min	15–20 min	2–4 min
FDA approval	2008	2012	Clinical evaluation

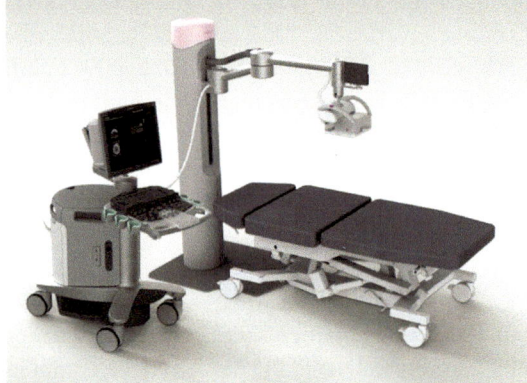

Fig. 1.1 US device for automated breast volume scanning ACUSON S2000 ABVS

standard mammography compression paddle. 3D automated systems were approved in the USA and Europe to conduct screening studies in 2012 for breast cancer detection as an adjunct to mammography and for screening symptom-free women with increased density of the breast tissue who had not previously undergone surgery. In clinics in Europe and the USA, a uniform protocol for the computer-aided study of mammary glands is used, consisting of three consecutive scans of each breast (one in the coronal plane and two in oblique planes). Each automated scan lasts an average of 1 min. The transducer paddle is placed over the breast with a small amount of compression applied to stabilize the breast. Depending on the size of the breast, more than one scan may be required to cover the entire field of interest. The average total time to complete the

examination is 15 min. Unification allows standardized breast images to be obtained regardless of the experience and qualifications of the physician or staff, and unlike HHUS, the examination can be performed by trained technologists, which is relevant for the USA because it reduces the workload on the physician. After acquisition the ABVS 3D data are stored on the hard disk of the device and then transferred to a special workstation for further interpretation and analysis.

Other types of hardware combined study systems with the transducer fixed in a special couch and with a prone patient position. The scanning is performed in a rotational manner, with a transducer configured for circumferential data acquisition. The sensor has a concave shape and rotates 360°. This system can be combined with MRI data for a more detailed representation of the breast status, for example, by using virtual sonography technology (US/MRI). Currently, this technology is under development and being studied in clinical trials and is yet to be approved.

In the future, the two fundamentally different physical principles of imaging will be integrated: 3D US and digital breast tomosynthesis. Currently, Siemens is developing methods of combining these image modalities in one study. This will allow the physician to obtain the maximum amount of diagnostic information in the minimum time. This technology is not yet available on the market, there is only a prototype of the future system, and tests are being conducted on phantoms. The results of testing this system on phantoms were first presented at the European

Congress of Radiology in 2015. There is no doubt that this method will be superior to ABVS and DBT alone and will identify breast pathologies with a greater degree of certainty.

Automation significantly reduces the time of a patient examination and helps reduce the subjectivity of the US data, which can provide significant advantages in screening programs. The high quality of images from modern diagnostic systems increases the sensitivity of the US method in detecting cancer.

Literature

1. Jackson VP, Kelly-Fry E, Rothschild PA et al (1986) Automated breast sonography using a 7.5-MHz PVDF transducer: preliminary clinical evaluation. Work in progress. Radiology 159:679–684
2. Maturo VG, Zusmer NR, Gilson AJ et al (1980) Ultrasound of the whole breast utilizing a dedicated automated breast scanner. Radiology 137:457–463
3. Chou YH, Tiu CM, Chen J et al (2007) Automated full-field breast ultrasonography: the past and the present. J Med Ultrasound 15:31–44
4. Shin HJ, Kim HH, Cha JH (2015) Current status of automated breast ultrasonography. Ultrasonography 34(3):165–172
5. Food US, Administration D (2012) Medical devices: Somo-V Automated Breast Ultrasound System (ABUS): P110006 [Internet]. U.S. Food and Drug Administration, Silver Spring
6. Kelly KM, Dean J, Comulada WS et al (2010) Breast cancer detection using automated whole breast ultrasound and mammography in radiographically dense breasts. Eur Radiol 20:734–742
7. Kaplan SS (2014) Automated whole breast ultrasound. Radiol Clin North Am 52:539–546
8. Kelly KM, Richwald GA (2011) Automated whole-breast ultrasound: advancing the performance of breast cancer screening. Semin Ultrasound CT MR 32:273–280

ABVS technology is being actively studied for cancer examination both as a screening technology and as replacement for HHUS as an automatic method. Most publications have compared the performance of ABVS and HHUS. The second most frequent are studies of the opinions of experts on certain BI-RADS-specified characteristics of breast masses described by the two methods. Currently, data is being accumulated on mass screening programs using ABUS technology. Only a few publications discuss the scanning technique. And even fewer articles analyze the comparability of tumor size measured by ABVS with the findings of surgery.

Kelly et al. [1] performed a multicenter prospective study of 4419 women with dense glandular tissue and/or risk of breast cancer development. They compared the capabilities of mammography in combination with semiautomatic whole-breast ultrasound (WBUS) and other radiological techniques [1]. This work showed promising results. An additional 3.6 cancers detected per 1,000 women screened were reported, and these results are consistent with the recommendations of the American College of Radiology [1]. The sensitivity of semiautomatic WBUS as a single method was 67% (38/57) and of mammography alone was 40% (23/57); however, with the combined approach, the sensitivity increased to 81% (46/57). According to the data, automated whole-breast ultrasound doubles the cancer detection rate and triples the identification of invasive cancers sized less than 1 cm [1].

Kelly et al. [2] also analyzed radiologists' performance for cancer detection in women with dense glandular tissue using ABUS. They found that the radiologists were able to improve cancer detection with an increase of 63% in the callbacks of cancer cases and only a 4% decrease in the correct identification of true-negative cases. They concluded that ABUS will play a significant role in the screening of women with dense breast tissue [2].

Golatta et al. [3] studied 983 patients and 1966 breasts. On the basis of biopsies carried out in the USA, they reported a high predictive value of a negative test result, which was 98% (1520/1551 cases), with high specificity of 85% (1794/1520) and sensitivity of 74% (88/119). Therefore they suggested that ABUS could be a promising method for breast studies, especially in screening programs [3]. This is the basic study assessing the possibilities of the method based on pathologic morphology.

Table 2.1 presents the main studies and conclusions obtained by the authors during ABUS [1–7].

According to numerous studies, ABVS is not inferior to conventional handheld US in detection and differential diagnosis of breast neoplasms while also exceeding it in some features. The informative value of ABVS is equivalent to HHUS in describing mass features and final assessment according to BI-RADS.

In 2011, Shin HJ et al. studied 55 women with 145 breast masses [4]. Five radiologists with varying experience detected from 74 to 88% of

© Springer International Publishing Switzerland 2017
V. Gazhonova, *3D Automated Breast Volume Sonography*, DOI 10.1007/978-3-319-41971-8_2

Table 2.1 Analysis of the publications on automatic breast volume sonography

Author	Study type	Number of patients	Ultrasound scanner	Summary
Kelly et al. [1]	Screening	4.419	Hybrid system SonoCine	ABUS doubles overall cancer detection and triples detection of 1 cm-or-less invasive cancers
Kelly et al. [2]	Screening	102	Hybrid system SonoCine	ABUS in addition to mammography reduces the frequency of callback rates in women with dense breast
Shin et al. [4]	Diagnostic	55	3D ABVS Acuson S2000	ABVS can identify masses larger than 1.2 cm and demonstrates substantial agreement for lesion description and final assessment
Wojcinski et al. [6]	Diagnostic	100	3D ABVS Acuson S2000	ABVS shows a high sensitivity (83 %) and fair interobserver concordance ($k=0.36$). ABVS has a high number of false-positive results
Chae et al. [12]	Diagnostic	58	3D ABVS Acuson S2000	ABVS allows identification of additional masses, detected by breast MRI, and may play a role as a replacement tool for handheld second-look US
Golatta et al. [3]	Mixed	983	Somo-V 3D ABUS	ABUS shows a high NPV (98 %), a high specificity (85 %), and a high sensitivity (74 %) (all cases confirmed by US-guided biopsy)

ABVS automatic breast volume sonography, *ABUS* automated breast ultrasound, *NPV* negative predictive value, *US* ultrasonography, *HHUS* handheld ultrasound

the masses; substantial agreement was reached on the description of the mass features ($k=0.61-0.72$) and BI-RADS final assessment category ($k=0.63$). According to the study, ABVS can identify masses larger than 1.2 cm in 92.0 % of cases.

According to the recent publication of Golatta et al. [3], with analysis of 84 ABVS breast cancer examinations in 42 women by six breast diagnostic specialists unaware of the results of breast imaging and medical history, it was revealed that agreement of ABVS examination to HHUS, mammography, and pathology was fair to substantial depending on the specific analysis

kappa value for all lesions ($k=0.35$). Agreement improved when dichotomizing the interpretation into benign (BI-RADS 1,2) and suspicious (BI-RADS 4,5)—kappa value −0.52 [5]. Wojcinski S et al. in 2011 and in 2013 obtained the same results for interobserver concordance ($k=0.36$). And with respect to the true category, the conditional inter-rate validity coefficient was kappa −0.18 for benign cases and kappa −0.80 for malignant cases. The likelihood of missing cancer in this method is very low. The authors concluded that ABVS examination in addition to mammography alone could detect a relevant number of previously occult breast cancers.

However, the method had a high number of false-positive results, with a rate of second-look ultrasounds of up to 48.8 % [6].

The first work by Wojcinski et al. [7] provided data on the one hand promising and on the other hand ambiguous for ABVS diagnostic performance and interobserver concordance: sensitivity (100 %), limited accuracy of the method (66 %), and dubious specificity (52.8 %) [7]. In subsequent work [6], the sensitivity of ABVS reduced to 83 %, and the number of false-positive results increased. The authors considered the differences in expert opinion relative to the character and nature of the masses when using ABVS as significant. They consider that this method is not yet ready to be employed for screening [6].

Despite this, in the USA and Canada, this method is positioned as a screening method to be used in women in a risk group for breast cancer. The authors of the study ACRIN 6666 described the following potential benefits of ABUS as a screening method in comparison with conventional US: standardization while conducting the ultrasound study, reduced operator dependence, and saving the physician's time [8]. And in Europe researchers consider the method as the best in women with already identified masses in the BI-RADS 3, 4, and 5 score group, to exclude or confirm signs of malignancy. Despite high accuracy, ABVS must still be regarded as an experimental technique for conclusion, which definitely needs further evaluation studies, as conducted by Wojcinski in 2011 [1]. The multicenter study by Lander et al. in 2011 evaluated the importance of ABVS as compared to conventional HHUS to identify masses in breast cancer screening programs [9]. According to numerous data, ABVS missed none of the breast cancers studied [10, 11]. Also, ABVS allows identification of additional masses and can replace HHUS in repeated ultrasound examinations [12].

Thus, the use of ABVS only for cancer identification in breasts provides a high sensitivity of examination, reaching 83–100 %. This will maximize the specificity and precision of ABVS in identifying cancer in a specially selected group of women, for example, with BI-RADS types 4 and 5.

Comparative studies of ABVS and HHUS for differentiation of benign and malignant breast lesions showed similarity or superiority of diagnostic accuracy of ABVS in numerous papers (Table 2.2) [13, 22–25]. Wang and Chen [13, 14] reported that ABVS is a promising modality for the clinical diagnosis of breast masses with retraction phenomenon and hyperechoic rim in the coronal plane, although the modalities do not differ in accuracy for the differentiation of breast masses; in a study of 81 patients by Lin et al. [15], ABVS and HHUS exhibited high sensitivity (both 100 %) and high specificity (95.0 % and 85.0 %, respectively). This high sensitivity of the method is enabled by the identifying of the "retraction" phenomenon on the coronal plane. This phenomenon, according to Lin et al., has 100 % specificity, 80 % sensitivity, and 91.4 % accuracy in differentiating benign and malignant breast masses [15]. The authors concluded that automated breast volume scanning is a promising modality in breast imaging; it provides advantages of better lesion size prediction, operator independence, and visualization of the whole breast. Another interesting work was that of Xu et al. [17] in which they evaluated the role of both ABVS and US elastography. They reported that both methods showed substantial interobserver reliability and the combined use of ABVS and US elastography was useful in improving diagnostic accuracy and specificity.

Whang [16] published data on 153 patients with 165 lesions and reported no significant differences between ABVS and HHUS with a slight diagnostic advantage of ABVS.

ABVS is advantageous as compared with HHUS in that it is less dependent on the examiners, has excellent reproducibility, and can determine the location of lesions more accurately by obtaining images of the overall breast.

With regard to malignancy based on the BI-RADS categories that is solely dependent on ABVS, Tozaki and Fukuma [18] showed similar results to HHUS; the accuracy of both methods in detecting cancer was the same. Kim et al. reported that there was substantial interobserver agreement in the final assessment of solid BI-RADS categories 4 and 5 breast masses using ABVS and HHUS [19].

Table 2.2 Comparison of the diagnostic value of HHUS vs ABVS in differential diagnosis between benign and malignant breast masses

Author, year	Number of patients/ masses identified	Precision, % (2D vs 3D)	Sensitivity, % (2D vs 3D)	Specificity, % (2D vs 3D)	Conclusion
Wang et al. 2012 [13]	213/239	85.3 vs 85.8	90.6 vs 95.3	80.5 vs 82.5	Diagnostic performance of both methods is similar
Chen et al. 2013 [14]	175/219	87.2 vs 88.1	88 vs 92.5	87.5 vs 86.2	Diagnostic performance of both methods is the same
Lin et al. 2012 [15]	81/95	91.4 vs 97.1	100 vs 100	85 vs 95	Diagnostic performance of ABVS is higher than that of HHUS
Whang et al. 2012 [16]	153/165	91.5 vs 94.5	93.2 vs 96.1	88.7 vs 91.9	Diagnostic performance of ABVS is higher than that of HHUS. ABVS is a promising method in the study of the breast
Xu et al. 2014 [17]	41/no data	Sonoelastography +ABVS 95.7	100%	87.5	The combination of ABVS and elastography increases the diagnostic performance of the examination

Li et al. [26], after reviewing 33 cases of DCIS and comparing them with the histopathology data, concluded that ABVS appears to assess the extent of pure ductal carcinoma in situ (DCIS) better than HHUS and can provide more accurate information pre-operation.

ABVS has a shorter examination time than HHUS. The average scanning time of ABVS, as Kim et al. [19] reported, was 9.8 ± 1.3 min, while the average scanning time of HHUS was 19.6 ± 1.6 min (data not shown). According to the authors, ABVS has certain advantages for the examination of masses located behind the nipple. They used the four-scan technique, as recommended in a number of other works [19].

Chang et al. [20] have shown that the frequency of detection of occult cancer after mammography is lower for ABVS than for HHUS, that is, 35.5 % vs 48.8 %, and some experience and training are required to improve image analysis skills with ABVS.

A number of works are devoted to studying scanning techniques. Thus, in the work of Tozaki et al., 2010, the per-quadrant scanning technique is described, with analysis of four areas: the upper-outer, lower-outer, upper-inner, and lower-inner quadrants [21]. The same technology was suggested by Isobe et al., for the study of the retroareolar area [22]. But regardless of the scanning technique, ABVS imaging was inferior to handheld US for detecting breast lesions under the nipple. Zhang et al. use the three-scan technique for ABVS: coronal, lateral, and medial [23]. Other authors performed a standard three-scan technique.

The standard recommended examination technique includes three slices: coronal (craniocaudal), mediolateral, and latero-medial. In this way, not all the tomographic slices of the breast can be correlated with the X-ray mammographic image. We believe that ABVS and mammography should operate as two complementary and not independent methods.

We suggest a 3D data collection methodology [24]. We added direct upper-lower quadrant slices to the mediolateral or latero-medial. This allows two orthogonal views of ABVS images for comparison with those of standard mammography views. Automatic breast volume sonography followed mammography in most of the patients after 40 years to clarify the changes identified and to search for or to give precise topography of the additional pathological masses. Manifestations of breast cancer are so diverse that only a comprehensive examination with mammography as the first stage and US as the second stage, with one technique complementing the other, allows evaluation of a specific set of symptoms indicating breast malignancy. No variants of patient positioning during 3D examination were found in the literature similar to ours. We revealed a high correlation coefficient of the ACR BI-RADS breast types with 100 % diagnostic accuracy between ABVS and mammography. In addition, ABVS, according to our study, has improved the sensitivity of mammography in detecting cancer in patients with dense breast [25].

So, sufficient experience has already accumulated worldwide in the application of 3D automatic scanning technology. Despite the variations in diagnostic performance of the method, researchers agree that the ABVS technique is undeniably promising and additional studies are needed of outstanding issues and scanning technology. Further work needs to concentrate on determination of mass diagnosis accuracy and evaluation of performance in screening programs in multicenter studies.

Literature

1. Kelly KM, Dean J, Comulada WS et al (2010) Breast cancer detection using automated whole breast ultrasound and mammography in radiographically dense breasts. Eur Radiol 20:734–742
2. Kelly KM, Dean J, Lee SJ et al (2010) Breast cancer detection: radiologists' performance using mammography with and without automated whole-breast ultrasound. Eur Radiol 20:2557–2564
3. Golatta M, Baggs C, Schweitzer-Martin M, Domschke C, Schott S, Harcos A et al (2015) Evaluation of an automated breast 3D-ultrasound system by comparing it with hand-held ultrasound (HHUS) and mammography. Arch Gynecol Obstet 291:889–895
4. Shin HJ, Kim HH, Cha JH et al (2011) Automated ultrasound of the breast for diagnosis: interobserver agreement on lesion detection and characterization. AJR Am J Roentgenol 197:747–754
5. Golatta M, Franz D, Harcos A et al (2013) Interobserver reliability of automated breast volume scanner (ABVS) interpretation and agreement of ABVS findings with hand held breast ultrasound (HHUS), mammography and pathology results. Eur J Radiol 13(8):332–336
6. Wojcinski S, Gyapong S, Farrokh A et al (2013) Diagnostic performance and inter-observer concordance in lesion detection with the automated breast volume scanner (ABVS). BMC Med Imaging 13:36
7. Wojcinski S, Farrokh A, Hille U et al (2011) The automated breast volume scanner (ABVS): initial experiences in lesion detection compared with conventional handheld B-mode ultrasound: a pilot study of 50 cases. Int J Womens Health 13:337–346
8. ACR practice guideline for the performance of a breast ultrasound examination (2011) American College of Radiology. Revised 2011 (Resolution 11) [Internet]. American College of Radiology, Reston
9. Lander MR, Tabar L (2011) Automated 3-D breast ultrasound as a promising adjunctive screening tool for examining dense breast tissue. Semin Roentgenol 46:302–308
10. Wenkel E, Heckmann M, Heinrich M et al (2008) Automated breast ultrasound: lesion detection and BI-RADS classification – a pilot study. Rofo 180:804–808
11. Jacobs OE, Rozhkova NI, Maso ML et al (2014) The experience of breast virtual sonography. Ann Roentgenol Radiol 1:23–32 (article in Russian)
12. Chae EY, Shin HJ, Kim HJ et al (2013) Diagnostic performance of automated breast ultrasound as a replacement for a hand-held second-look ultrasound for breast lesions detected initially on magnetic resonance imaging. Ultrasound Med Biol 39:2246–2254
13. Wang HY, Jiang YX, Zhu QL (2012) Differentiation of benign and malignant breast lesions: a comparison between automatically generated breast volume scans and handheld ultrasound examinations. Eur J Radiol 81(11):3190–3200
14. Chen L, Chen Y, Diao XN et al (2013) Comparative study of automated breast 3-D ultrasound and hand held B-mode ultrasound for differentiation of benign and malignant breast masses. Ultrasound Med Bio 139(10):1735–1742
15. Lin X, Wang J, Han F et al (2012) Analysis of eighty-one cases with breast lesions using automated breast volume scanner and comparison with handheld ultrasound. Eur J Radiol 13(5):873–878
16. Wang ZL, Xw JH, Li JL et al (2012) Comparison of automated breast volume scanning to hand-held ultrasound and mammography. Radiol Med 13(8):1287–1293

17. Xu C, Wei S, Xie Y (2014) Combined use of the auto-
    mated breast volume scanner and the US elastogra-
    phy for the differentiation of benign from malignant
    lesions of the breast. BMC Cancer 14:798
18. Tozaki M, Fukuma E (2010) Accuracy of determin-
    ing preoperative cancer extent measured by auto-
    mated breast ultrasonography. Jpn J Radiol 13(10):
    771–773
19. Kim YW, Kim SK, Youn HJ et al (2013) The clini-
    cal utility of automated breast volume scanner: a pilot
    study of 139 cases. J Breast Cancer 16(3):329–334
20. Chang JM, Moon WK, Cho N et al (2011) Breast can-
    cers initially detected by hand-held ultrasound: detec-
    tion performance of radiologists using automated
    breast ultrasound data. Acta Radiol 52:8–14
21. Tozaki M, Isobe S, Yamaguchi M et al (2010) Optimal
    scanning technique to cover the whole breast using
    an automated breast volume scanner. Jpn J Radiol
    28(4):325–328
22. Isobe S, Tozaki M, Yamaguchi M et al (2011)
    Detectability of breast lesions under the nipple using
    an automated breast volume scanner: comparison

with handheld ultrasonography. Jpn J Radiol 13(5):
    361–365
23. Zhang Q, Hu B, Hu B et al (2012) Detection of breast
    lesions using an automated breast volume scanner
    system. J Int Med Res 40(1):300–306
24. Gazhonova VE, Bachurina EM, Khlustina EM et al
    (2014) Automatic sonotomography of mammary
    glands (3D ABVS). Part 1. Integration of ABVS
    method in the radiological imaging standards.
    Polyclinic. Radiology 42–48 (article in Russian)
25. Gazhonova VE, Efremova MP, Bachurina EM et al
    (2015) The possibilities of assessing the glandular
    type of the breast structure by sonotomography from
    the standpoint of the risk factor for breast cancer
    development. Ann Roentgenol Radiol 5:23–29 (arti-
    cle in Russian)
26. Li N, Jiang YX, Zhu QL et al (2013) Accuracy of
    an automated breast volume ultrasound system for
    assessment of the pre-operative extent of pure ductal
    carcinoma in situ: comparison with a conventional
    handheld ultrasound examination. Ultrasound Med
    Biol 39:2255–2263

3.1 Indications

In our view the main indication for ABVS should be dense breast tissue. In patients with fatty degeneration, the prevailing method is mammography.

ABVS should be used for supplemental screening after MMG in doubtful diagnostic cases or if masses or groups of microcalcifications were detected. When the lesion is evident on a mammogram, the topographic diagnosis is established with ABVS in relevant slices. Conversely, all local changes identified during ABVS could be projected on a mammogram, defining the characteristic radiographic features of the masses.

Reproducibility, the possibility of delayed interpretation, and second-look readings in automatic breast volume sonography provide unlimited opportunities for examiner-independent monitoring of benign masses.

A higher level of comfort for patients with breast implants is provided during ABVS examination compared to traditional mammography systems due to minimal breast compression during the study.

One of the major advantages of ABVS over other radiological methods (mammography and MRI) is that the images are produced with the patient in a supine position, similar to that for breast surgery. Therefore, the coronal slices can be used for surgical planning. These images are more easily interpreted not only by radiologists but also by surgeons.

Despite some difficulties in the scanning of patients with macromastia, we believe that this condition is also an indication for ABVS. Additional slices of the lower and mediolateral quadrants and special patient positioning during the examination allow the whole breast to be examined in macromastia cases.

To summarize, the indications for ABVS are the following:

- Exclusion or confirmation of cancer signs in BI-RADS 3–5 lesions, detected by US or MMG in women with dense breast
- As a screening method for young women with a high risk of breast cancer
- Documentation of multifocality or multicentricity of BI-RADS 5 and 6 tumors
- To follow up benign tumors
- Postoperatively to identify the glandular structure
- To clarify the topography of masses before biopsy or surgery

The potential indications for a more expanded ABVS study could be detection of cancer in young patients with a high risk of breast cancer, detection of multicentricity and multifocality of tumors (especially DCIS), study of the contralateral breast with existing breast cancer (in a hereditary disease, the risk of contralateral breast cancer reaches 65 %), detection of a residual tumor after lumpectomy, identification of occult breast cancer (when regional or distant metastases were found,

© Springer International Publishing Switzerland 2017
V. Gazhonova, *3D Automated Breast Volume Sonography*, DOI 10.1007/978-3-319-41971-8_3

in cases of MMG-negative or HHUS-negative tumors), precise estimation of tumor size (in a radiographically dense breast, in lobular carcinoma, in tumors with an extensive intraductal component, or, DCIS, if a lesion spreads in the surrounding tissue), and follow-up of the tumor during neoadjuvant chemotherapy before surgery.

Currently, the precise definition of the indications and risk groups for clinically and economically justified use of ABVS remains unclear. Also the screening interval for this group of patients and the optimal screening starting age are yet to be determined.

3.2   Technical Background

The ACUSON S2000 ABVS is an ultrasound system that includes an ultrasound scanner and a special stationary device with transducer attached to a mechanical arm (Fig. 3.1). The 14L5BV transducer (maximum frequency 14 MHz, average scanning frequency 10 MHz, width of 15.4 cm, 768 piezoelectric elements) receives the image of the entire breast volume in 1 min with a maximum depth of up to 6 cm. During the automatic collection of 3D data, 16.8 cm distance is covered, acquiring 318 high-resolution slices for post-processing (resolution: axial 0.09 mm, lateral 0.16 mm, and sagittal 0.44 mm).

In order to optimize the ABVS results, there is a wide range of known imaging modes including tissue harmonic imaging (THI), AdvancedSieClear™ spatial compounding, and Dynamic TCE™ (tissue contrast enhancement) technology, as well as new processing algorithms for nipple shadow and reverberation artifacts that are automatically applied when using the ABVS. The reverberation removal algorithm processes the 3D data and determines whether tissue contact is present and where it is not. The data corresponding to the area with no tissue contact are removed. This is intended to suppress reverberation artifacts from the noncontact areas. The adaptive nipple shadow reduction tool analyzes data on a case-by-case basis and is thought to enhance the structures in the retroareolar area and to improve visualization of this important region. And finally, a gain collection algorithm analyzes the 3D data and adjusts for the brightness variation artifacts caused by transducer channel-to-channel effects.

A replaceable membrane is fixed to the transducer to ensure sufficient contact with the skin of the entire area. The patient is placed in the same position as for the HHUS. A special lotion that provides optimal imaging results is applied to the skin instead of the usual gel (Polysonic Ultrasound Lotion, Parker Laboratories, Inc, Fairfield, NJ). The transducer is positioned on the breast with slight pressure and locked prior to scanning (Fig. 3.2).

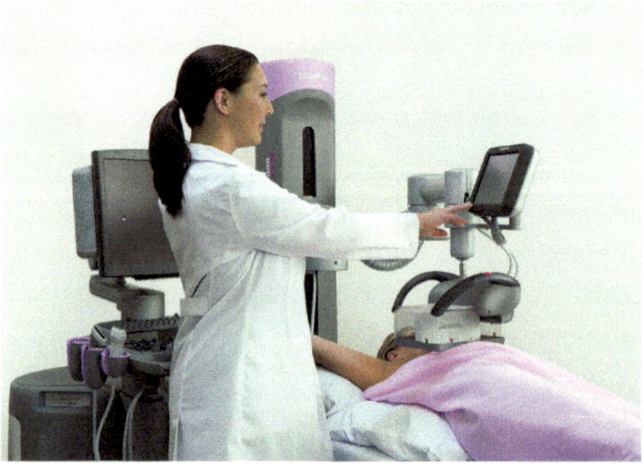

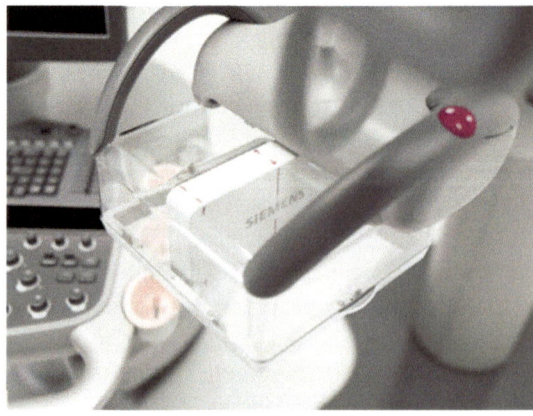

Fig. 3.1 US device for automated breast scanning. ACUSON S2000 ABVS

Fig. 3.2 Special linear transducer (14L5BV) for automatic volume scanning

The depth of scanning is specified from A to D (depending on the bra cup size), and then the scan area is selected: the right or the left breast (Fig. 3.3). The transducer is positioned on the breast according to the selected slices (R AP, R LAT, R MED, R SUP, R INF, R AXILLA, R OTHER or L AP, L LAT, L MED, L SUP, L INF, L AXILLA, L OTHER, corresponding to the ROI) as anterior-posterior, medial, lateral, upper, lower, axillary, and other, according to the proposed positions (Fig. 3.4).

Next, the scanning direction of the probe is selected by the button located on the transducer. The gathering of volume information may be performed upward or downward. Next stage is the acquisition of the 3D data. There is no need for the patient to hold her breath during the procedure. The probe is moved automatically in a given field, and at the end of the scan, it is automatically unlocked, so it can be removed from the gland. The automatic scanning procedure can be interrupted at any time by pressing the CANCEL button on the monitor screen.

3.3   Patient and Transducer Positions

We recommend the following special patient positioning for obtaining the ABVS slices.

3.3.1   AP Slice (Anteroposterior)

To obtain the slice, the patient is in a supine position with the ipsilateral hand behind the head. In this position the nipple is located centrally against

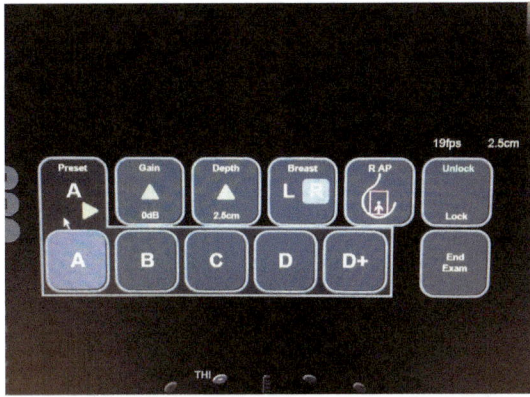

Fig. 3.3 The scanning parameters on the screen: depth, breast bra cup size, slice type

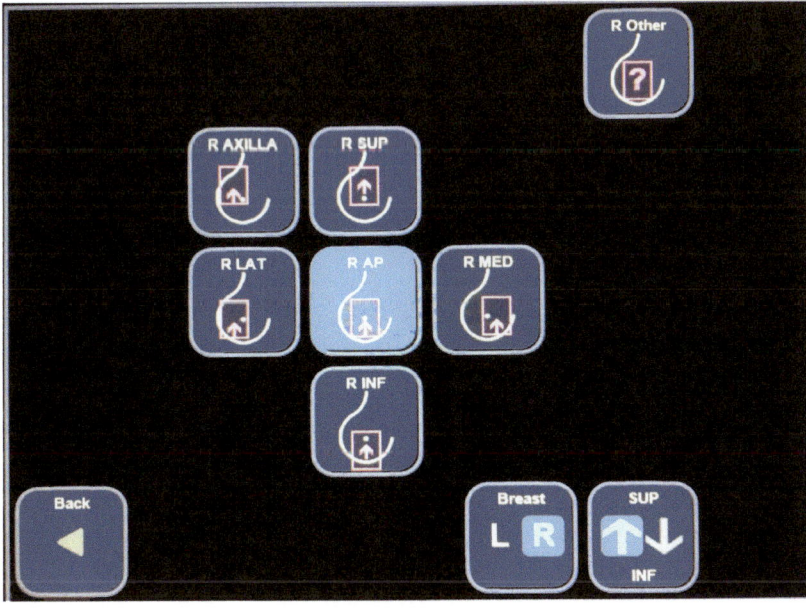

Fig. 3.4 The predefined positions of the scanner, with the number of standard slices for automatic scanning

the transducer where the arrow is, and the inner and outer quadrants of the breast are equidistant from it (Fig. 3.5). This is of major importance for precise further topographical measurements.

3.3.2 LAT Slice (Latero-Medial Oblique (LMO))

The technique for obtaining the slice is similar to that of mammography, but the patient is lying on her side, with the ipsilateral hand behind her head. The nipple area is shifted medially as far as possible from the scanning field to the edge of the scanning membrane being equidistant from the upper and lower quadrants. The lateral scanning

border of the transducer is marked with a red line (Fig. 3.6).

For the MED slice (*mediolateral oblique* (*MLo*)), the gland is shifted laterally to the side; the patient is in a supine position as during the AP slice with a maximum lateralization of the nipple in the scanning field (Fig. 3.7).

3.3.3 SUP Slice (Craniocaudal Superior-to-Inferior Slice)

To obtain this slice, it is necessary to raise the head of the couch in a slightly higher position with the ipsilateral arm lying close to the body. In severe breast ptosis, this maneuver is not needed.

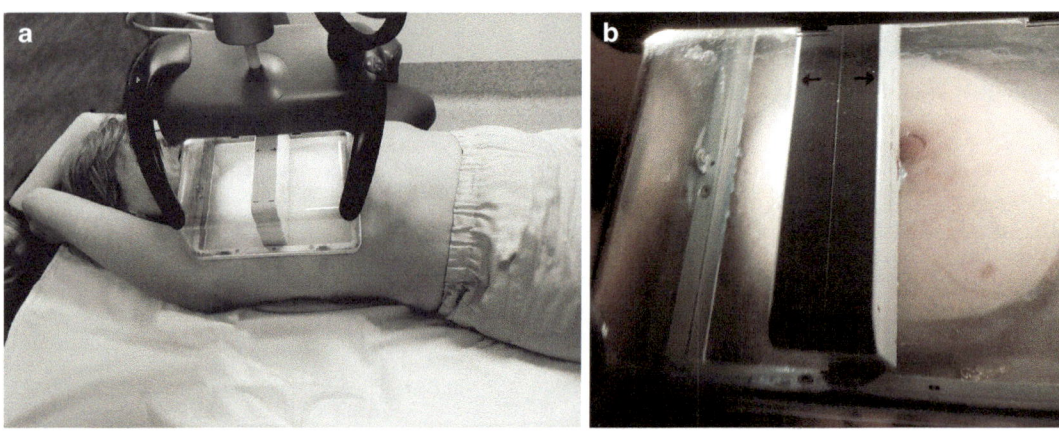

Fig. 3.5 Patient positioning and breast position while acquiring the coronal R AP slice. (**a**) Patient position during the ABVS study of the right breast. (**b**) Location of the breast under the transducer for an AP slice

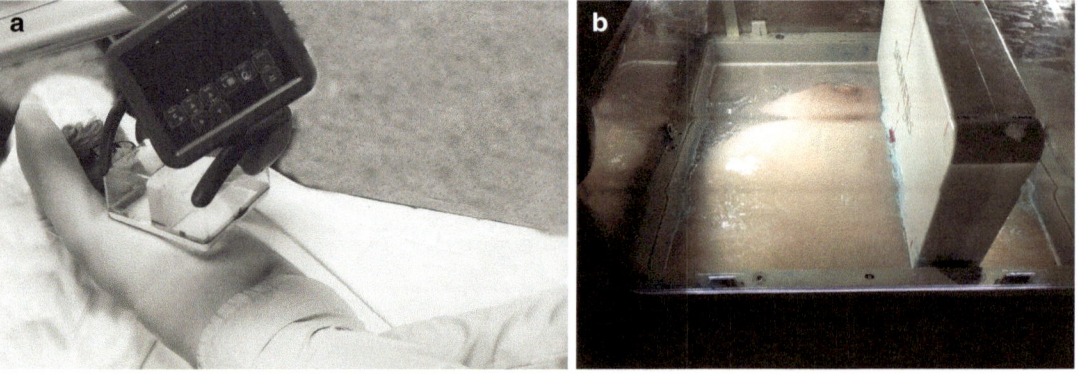

Fig. 3.6 Obtaining an R LAT slice (latero-medial oblique slice of the right breast). (**a**) Patient position during the ABVS exam. (**b**) Location of the breast under the transducer for an LMO slice

The transducer presses on the breast and shifts it downward to the chest. The nipple area in this position is displaced down from the scanning field, 1 cm from the membrane, centrally, so that inner and outer quadrants should be equidistant from the nipple (Fig. 3.8).

The INF slice (craniocaudal inferior-to-superior slice) is produced in the supine position, with the ipsilateral hand behind the head. The breast is shifted upward; the nipple is maximally displaced up the scanning membrane, 1 cm from the edge of the scanning field.

Maximum lateralization of the nipple in the mediolateral oblique (MED) or latero-medial oblique (LAT) and craniocaudal inferior-to-superior (INF) slices is applied to improve the

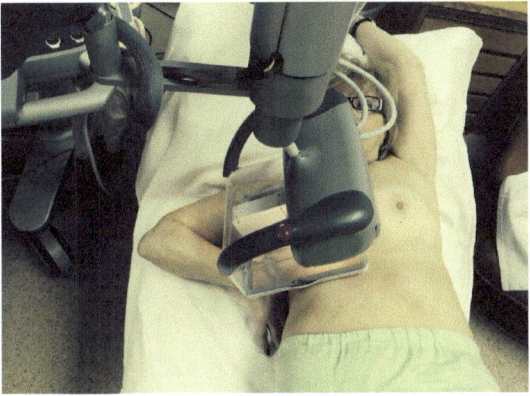

Fig. 3.7 Obtaining an R MED slice (mediolateral oblique slice of the right breast). Patient position

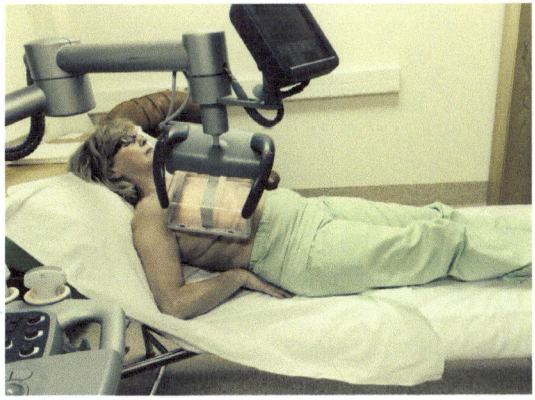

Fig. 3.8 Obtaining the R SUP (craniocaudal superior-to-inferior slice of the right breast). Patient position

visualization of the zone behind the nipple. If the lesions are located in the inner quadrant or in the lower quadrant, it is preferable to use the MED or INF slices instead of LAT or craniocaudal superior-to-inferior (SUP), respectively.

A pictogram of the performed slice is presented in the lower-left corner of the screen. This stage is used for selection of the best quality ABVS image series for storage. At this stage, the quantity, quality of the acquired information, adequacy, and necessity of additional scans are verified. It should be noted that the assessment of the quality of sonotomograms is important at this stage, as the patient is still in the examination room and the breast can be re-scanned with additional slices if necessary. During an automatic scan, motional or conversation artifacts arise in some cases, which adversely affect the perception of 3D data. Therefore, during the automatic scanning, the patient should not talk or move. Breathing chest movements do not interfere with scanning and do not alter the image. The lack of contact of the scanning membrane with the skin of the gland can cause some so-called "dark side" artifacts; this should be avoided. Unfortunately, it is difficult to achieve in some cases, e.g., in patients with breast scar deformation after breast conserving surgery or lumpectomy, in breast-expanders, in large tumors with nipple retraction, or, vice versa, with the bulging of the mass and, less often, after breast augmentation.

If the operator is satisfied with the information collected, he/she labels the position of the nipple, which allows orientation in the subsequent analysis, and confirms the saving of the collected information by pressing the SAVE button, and then all the data are stored. When the image is of poor quality, no saving is performed by clicking the REJECT button.

After the first slice, the US device automatically offers to acquire the next one, as programmed in the presets of the US scanner. On average, six standard slices are performed per patient. According to our recommendations for the use of the technology, it is necessary to perform the coronal, oblique latero-medial (or mediolateral), and craniocaudal superior-to-inferior slices of each gland. The number of slices depends on the size of the breast. The larger the breast, the more slices you need to perform. The more masses are examined; the more slices should be performed to fully collect all the information.

3.4   Image Analysis

After a particular scan is completed, the coronal plane of the acquired volume is displayed at skin level. This information is presented on the screen as a series of images that can be resliced from the top with the nipple down to the chest wall. The per-quadrant anatomy on ABVS scans

corresponds to the real location of the quadrants in the breast. The upper quadrants in all images using this technology are at the top of the scan, and the outer and inner quadrants correspond to the patient's position during the examination (Fig. 3.9).

Before collecting the next slice, quick preliminary topographical measurements could be performed for the entire volume produced on the screen. The image can be analyzed quickly by activating the *Advanced 3D* function on the monitor screen. It opens an extended menu for analysis of three-dimensional information. The most commonly used is two-view mapping mode. When an unclear object is selected on a cross

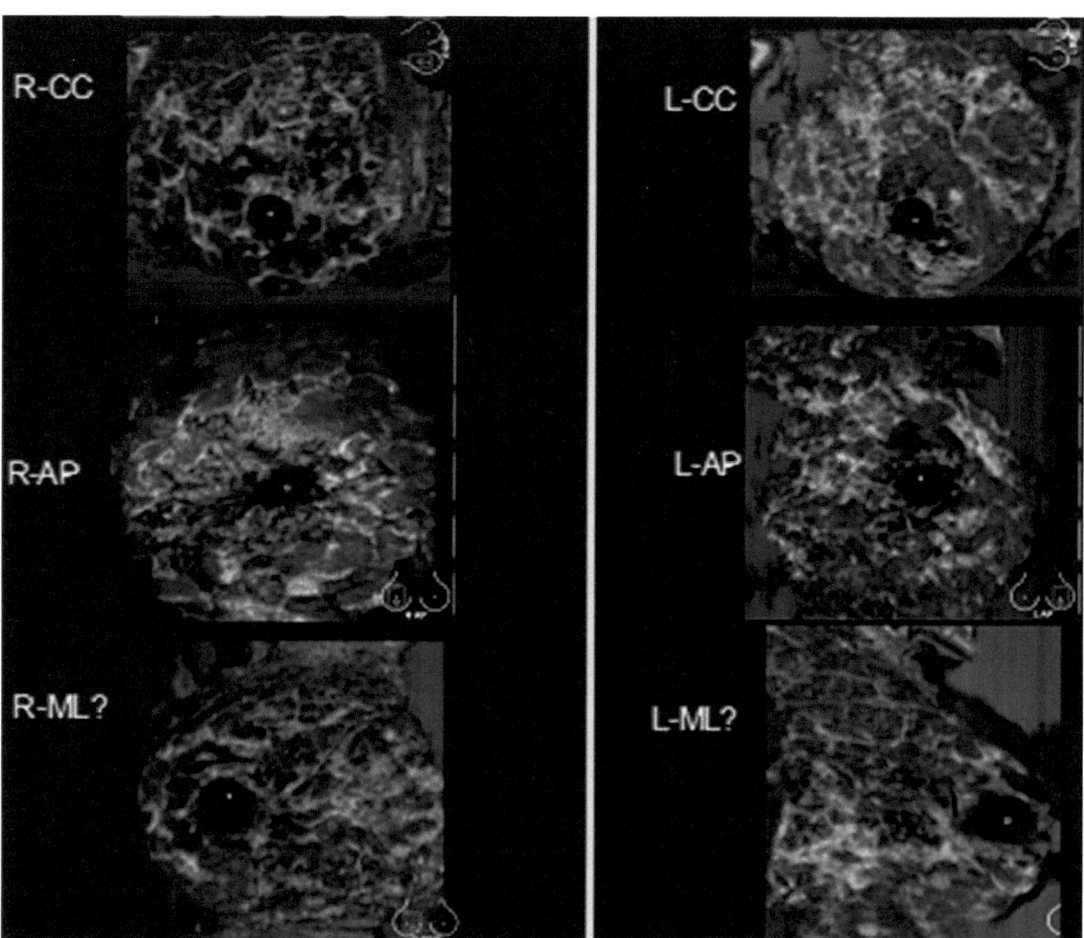

Fig. 3.9 US tomograms performed according to the technology under our recommendations. Right breast, three images; left breast, three images. Symbols: *R-CC*, right SUP slice; *L-CC*, left SUP slice; *R AP*, right anteroposterior coronal slice; *L AP*, left anteroposterior coronal slice; *R-ML*, right MED slice; and *L-ML*, left MED slice

section, the second part of the screen displays its coronal view. The left part of the screen shows the standard cross-sectional view of the mass of interest, and the right part of the screen shows the matching coronal slice (Fig. 3.10). Multislice analysis of the tumor can also be performed by specifying the slice thickness and desired plane. The US device allows the operator to set the required number of images on the screen during multislice viewing (Fig. 3.11). A cross-sectional view can be combined with multislice technology and provides data on a single picture (Fig. 3.12). The distance from the mass to the nipple, from the mass to the skin, or from the mass to the chest wall can also be measured. The entire breast structure is evaluated on the cine view; localization of lesions is clarified for quick appreciation of the pathology. There are plenty of choices for analysis of 3D data stored in the device.

This technique of acquiring 3D data in an ABVS examination provides comparability of ABVS images to mammograms. Standardization of the examination enables the reproducibility of subsequent follow-up images.

Finally, the entire set of volume scans is sent to a separate workstation for a deeper analysis and completing the final protocol. The processing is carried out on a special workstation (breast ultrasound review workstation) where the ABVS database is stored. After requesting the patient's file, the corresponding series are selected in the dialog box. All series are labeled with the appropriate R or L slice type (AP, LAT, MED, SUP, INF, AXILLA). All series of slices are presented in three mutually perpendicular planes. One can specify the view of the slices by the choice of icon in the monitor window.

Navigation is through each point being positioned on three axes X, Y, and Z (sagittal, coronal, and axial). The collected data is processed in arbitrary planes and slices, and ABVS tomograms of the breasts are generated which are comparable to those from RMG; topographical measurements are conducted in automatic mode by placing the cursor on the required object (Fig. 3.13).

Examination protocol and document selection standardization enable the matching of the symmetry of the structure of the right and left breasts, in the respective planes, and the reproducibility of the subsequent follow-up images with the same parameters and also the comparability with X-ray mammography data (Fig. 3.14).

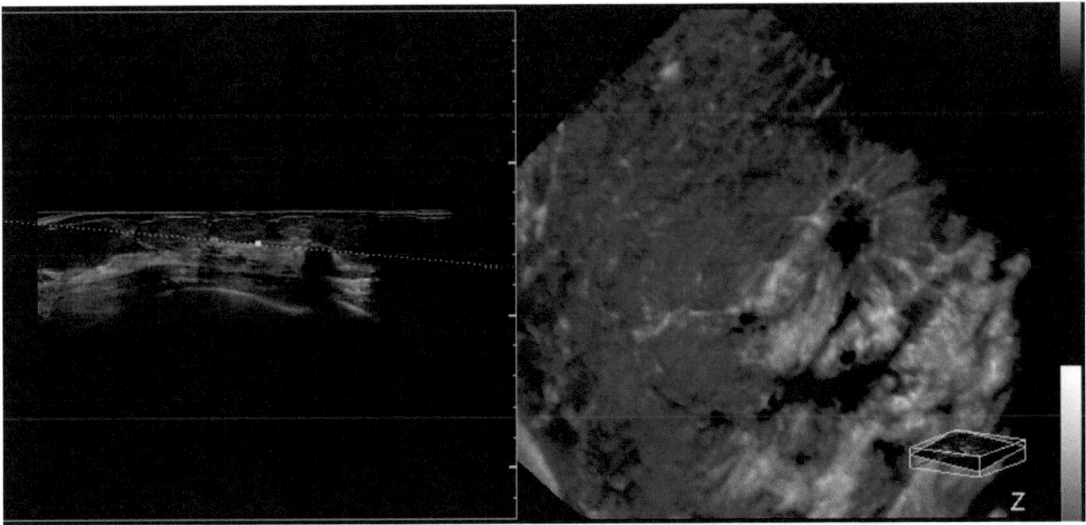

Fig. 3.10 Automated breast volume sonography of a breast lesion. There is an unclear hypoechoic mass with irregular shape on the left part, and on the right side, a coronal view of it is displayed. The lesion boundary is spiculated

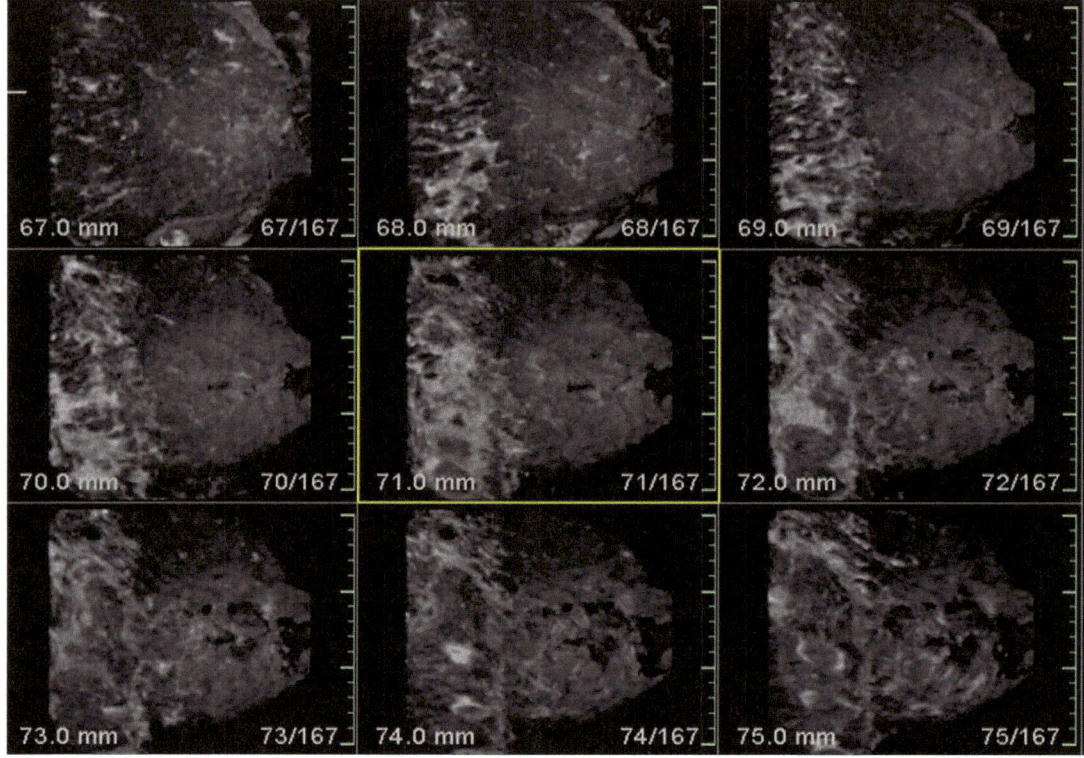

Fig. 3.11 ABVS with multislice image analysis. LAT slices with slice thickness of 1 mm. On the level of 70 mm (or the 70th of 167 slice images from the external part of the breast to the medial part), an area of structural impairment is clearly seen. It presented as a hypoechoic area with irregular margins, which starts from the nipple-areolar zone going deep into the glandular tissue. The breast conserving surgery confirmed invasive ductal carcinoma with invasion into the nipple

3.5   Protocols

The workstation (breast ultrasound review workstation) enables the generation of the protocol according to the BI-RADS classification automatically by clicking on the appropriate option in the operating window. It is possible to mark the mass of interest by requesting the relevant series of slices and marking the mass in them; the computer will automatically calculate its position: relative to the surface of the skin, relative to the nipple, and in relation to the clockface. All of these data and the image itself are automatically recorded in the protocol. The program does not limit the number of labeled masses. In the protocol the physician need only indicate the category of the mass by the 0–6 point classification. Pressing the PDF button, the final formation of the protocol starts in the ".pdf" format. The protocol contains information about the patient, labeled selected masses, all of their topographical characteristics, and the BI-RADS class, with an illustrative section (Fig. 3.15).

The protocol should be extended and complemented by information not included in the automatic computer version. The BI-RADS (Breast Imaging Report and Diagnosis) classification, referred to above, was first proposed for X-ray mammography and then for ultrasound. It contains information on the conditions of the examination, on the protocol, on the type of the gland, and on the class of the mass. The application of this classification is important for ABVS because it allows the selection of a group of patients for additional examination using this method. We offer a more advanced version of the protocol, which can be used as a template.

In the first section of the protocol (Fig. 3.16), the following personal data of the patient should be indicated: age, year of birth, menstrual

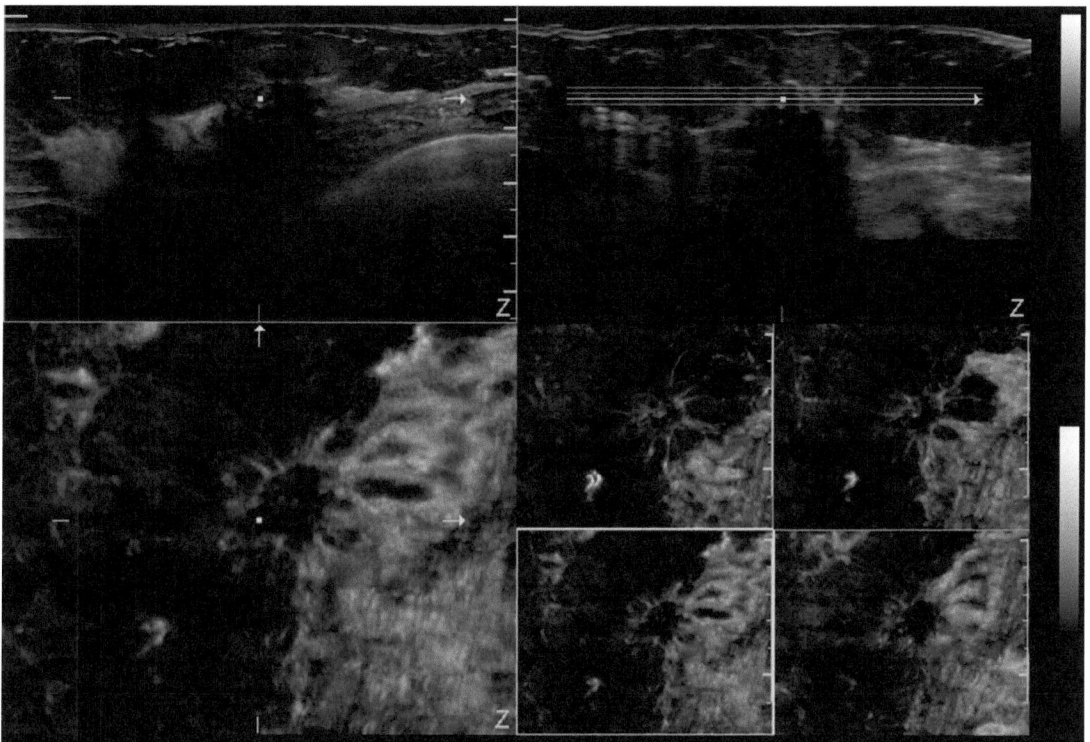

Fig. 3.12 ABVS images of the breast lesion (*upper left*, transverse plane; *upper right*, sagittal plane; *lower left*, coronal reconstruction; *lower right*, multislice view of the coronal scans). Thin slices are performed through the upper areas of the tumor, demonstrating the "spiculated" pattern on the coronal slice. The multislice view mode in the lower figures shows the relationship of the tumor with the anterior pectoralis fascia. The tumor has a tiny connection with the fascia that is clearly visible in the multislice view

function with indication of the day of the cycle, and information about combined oral (intrauterine) contraceptive treatment, if present. In the absence of the cycle, the following should be indicated: duration of menopause, information about hormone replacement, and other therapy that can affect the breast. Previous breast surgery and its type, with an indication of the quadrant and the side where the surgery was performed, should be included in the protocol.

The protocol further specifies the conditions of the study: method—ABVS and the equipment (ACUSON S2000 ABVS). Then all the completed views are listed with technical parameters and an indication of the depth of the slice. This is necessary for second-look and follow-up studies.

The protocol starts with a general assessment of the size and structure of the breasts (micromastia, normomastia, macromastia, pronounced ptosis, augmented breast). According to

the BI-RADS classification, four breast density types are described: ACR 1, ACR 2, ACR 3, and ACR 4 (1, 0 % of glandular tissue; 2, up to 25-50 % of glandular tissue; 3, more than 50 % but less than 75 % of glandular tissue; 4, absolutely dense gland, with more than 75 % glandular tissue). It is of great importance to indicate the distribution pattern of glandular tissue, depending on the age and physiological period, and the presence of asymmetries. The data should include information about the nipple-areolar zone, the nipple itself, pre- and retromammary space, pectoral fascia, and muscles. All the breast anatomy information should be compared and included in the protocol.

If pathological changes are detected, their type is defined according to BI-RADS classification, location, size, shape, contours, distal shadow intensity, and internal structure, and the presence of microcalcifications should be evaluated.

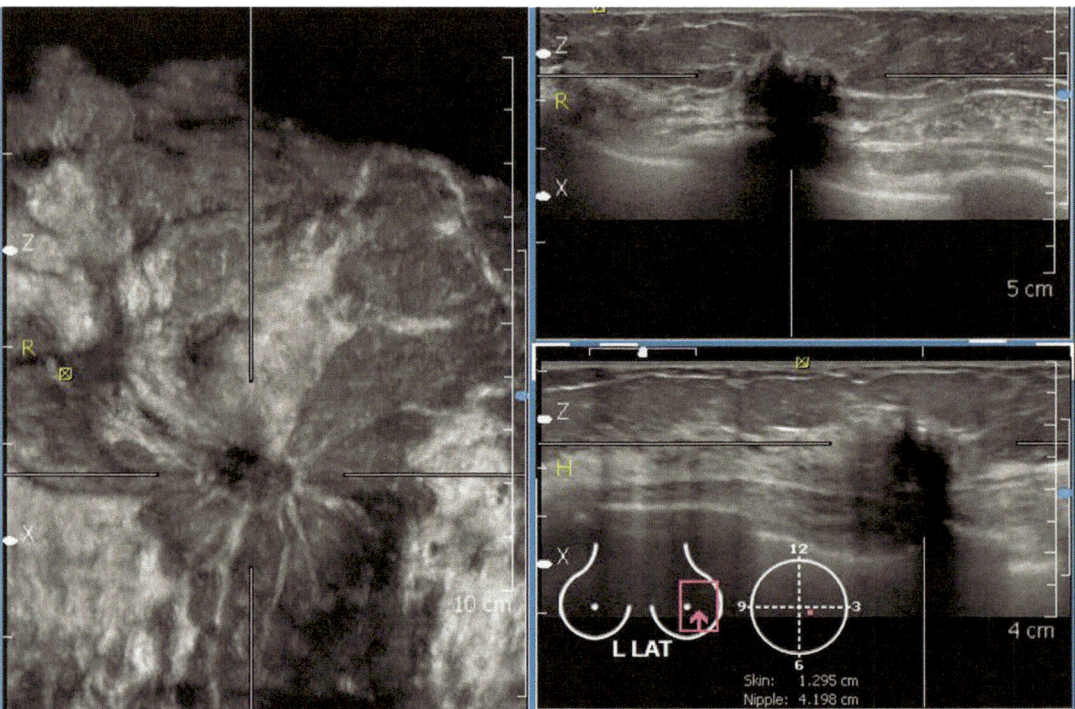

Fig. 3.13 ABVS images of the invasive ductal carcinoma of the breast from the workstation *(left*, coronal reconstruction; *upper right*, sagittal scan, *lower right*, transverse view). Multiplanar reconstruction of the tumor. On the left side of the figure, the mass is clearly visualized with a spiculated boundary. *L LAT*—left latero-medial view. A pictogram of the mass topography is presented in the bottom of the figure. The distance from the skin and from the nipple and clockface position of the tumor in the breast pictogram are shown. The point is visible at the 3 o'clock position where the tumor located

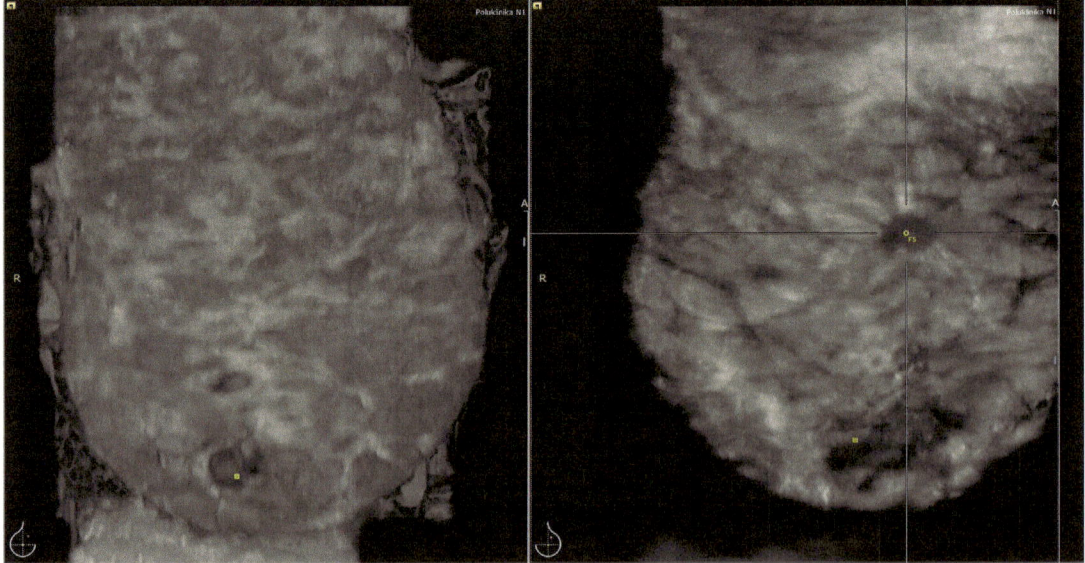

Fig. 3.14 *ABVS* image analysis on the workstation. The side-by-side comparison of consecutive slices of the right and left breasts. Craniocaudal SUP slices. The asymmetry of the structure is visible in both upper quadrants of the breast. In the right breast *(right part)*, an oval-shaped mass (fibroadenoma) is visible over the nipple. In the left breast *(left part)*, a long way from the nipple, a hypoechoic mass with retraction phenomenon is defined (The mass was pathologically confirmed as invasive ductal carcinoma)

Ultrasound Report:

Study Information		Report Summary
Patient	X	
Patient ID	14.11.28-14:19:59-DST-1.3.12.2.1107.5.5.2.208789	
Birth Date	12/23/65	**BI-RADS® Category: Highly suggestive of malignancy (BI-RADS® 5)**
Study	Breast	
Study Date	20141128	
Referring Physician		

Findings in this Study

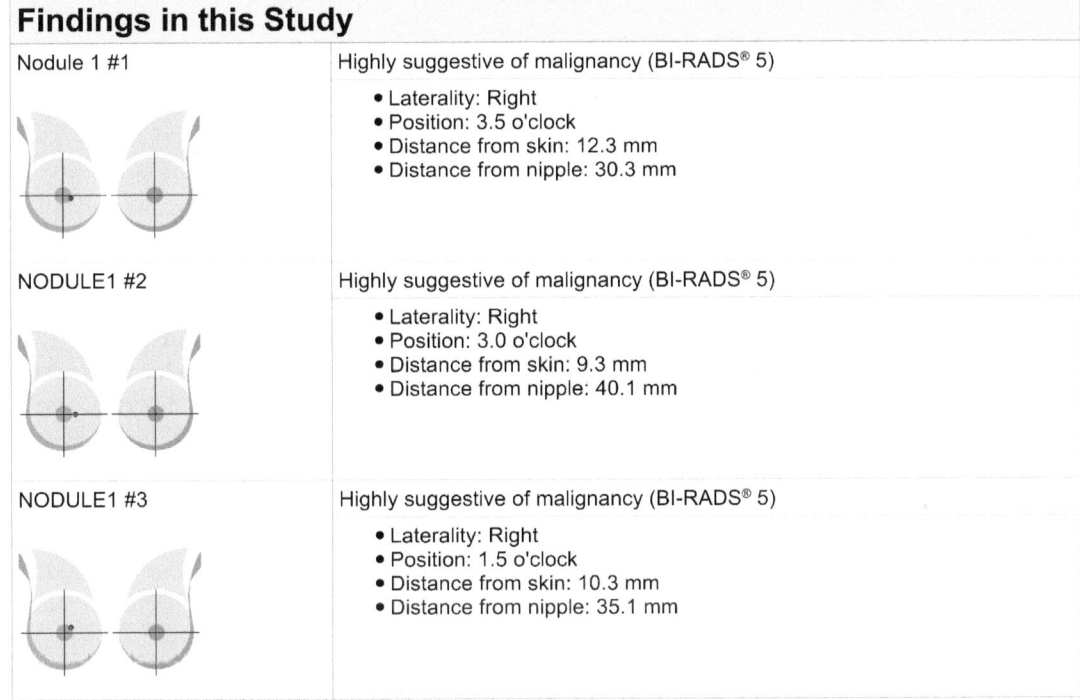

Nodule 1 #1	Highly suggestive of malignancy (BI-RADS® 5) • Laterality: Right • Position: 3.5 o'clock • Distance from skin: 12.3 mm • Distance from nipple: 30.3 mm
NODULE1 #2	Highly suggestive of malignancy (BI-RADS® 5) • Laterality: Right • Position: 3.0 o'clock • Distance from skin: 9.3 mm • Distance from nipple: 40.1 mm
NODULE1 #3	Highly suggestive of malignancy (BI-RADS® 5) • Laterality: Right • Position: 1.5 o'clock • Distance from skin: 10.3 mm • Distance from nipple: 35.1 mm

Fig. 3.15 Automatically generated protocol on a workstation according to the BI-RADS classification

3.6   Image Interpretation

Interpretation and analysis of any particular case consists of several stages: detection of the pathology and comparison of the changes with the reference method. Neither CT- nor MR-mammography images can be compared with MMG. Before ABVS it was impossible to correlate US data with MMG. This became possible only with the development of automated breast ultrasound and with

improvement of 3D technology. Despite the different physical principles, the images obtained by the two methods have many comparable characteristics. Both technologies use similar patient positioning and apply compression to the breast to produce a scan.

It is necessary to understand the possibilities and limitations of breast visualization by MMG and ABVS in order to perform good interpretation. It is worth mentioning that mammography

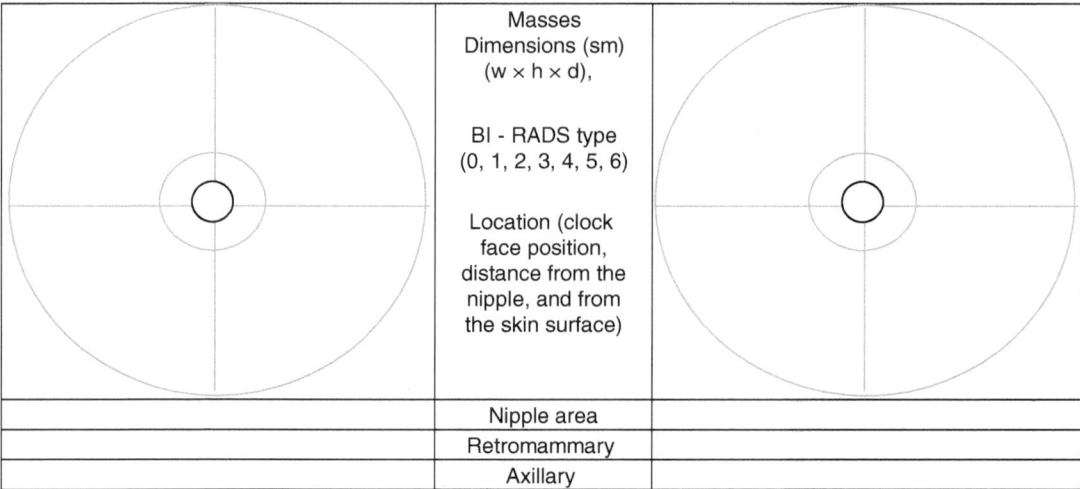

	Masses Dimensions (sm) (w × h × d), BI - RADS type (0, 1, 2, 3, 4, 5, 6) Location (clock face position, distance from the nipple, and from the skin surface)	
	Nipple area	
	Retromammary	
	Axillary	

Fig. 3.16 Advanced ABVS protocol on the ACUSON S2000 ABVS device

misses some areas of the breast, as they do not get covered by the field of view under the membrane: at the craniocaudal view, it is the upper-deep posterior portion of the breast and the axillary recess; in the LMO (latero-medial oblique) view, it is the medial-posterior area of the breast; and in the direct LM view, it is the posterior lateral portion of the gland [1]. The patient positioning and the acquisition technique in ABVS are slightly different from that in mammography. The breast is not compressed comparable to MMG but shifted and slightly pressed against the body by the transducer with attached paddle. Therefore, the areas of the gland that are not displayed on a mammogram are visible on ABVS. This is the main advantage and the complementary role of ABVS.

From all of the ABVS slices, the most suitable to compare with mammography views are the LAT and MED (mediolateral and latero-medial) and SUP (superior-to-inferior) views. They can be compared with the MLo and CC views on a mammography. These images in both ABVS and MMG provide clear visualization of the nipple, which serves as a topographical guide or matching point. The top or bottom contours of the breast are easily recognized by both technologies, which may be another landmark for matching. For comparing it is simply necessary to proportion the images on the top and bottom contours, placing the nipples into the center, and perform navigation.

Why should one perform this navigation with mapping projections? Firstly, not all of the shadow masses identified by MMG are malignant, and not all require verification using a needle biopsy. According to statistics, over 80 % of masses identified by MMG are benign [2, 3]. Projecting the image of an unclear mass from a mammogram on an ABVS tomogram, one can identify the nature of the mass more precisely (Figs. 3.17, 3.18, 3.19, and 3.20). In addition, this is, in our view, the greatest advantage of ABVS.

Secondly, the dense breast tissue on mammogram tumors could be negative and hide the symptoms of malignancy. If a combination of methods works together on one screen, these changes could be revealed more accurately, and many more tumors would be found at an early stage (Fig. 3.21). The preferable use of a combination of ABVS and MMG methods in breast screening has already been discussed in a number of works [4–8].

Both ABVS and MMG provide a pronounced contrasting of glandular and fatty tissue. The US shows fatty tissue as hypoechoic and glandular and fibrous ones as hyperechoic. American biophysics has shown that US can be used to measure breast density similar to mammography [9, 10]. The speeds of US wave propagation in different tissues differ reliably, and this difference can be determined by the human eye in the black-and-white scale spectrum. The ABVS wide aperture transducer allows one to capture a whole-breast gland in one scan and gives a picture of the whole gland in one image. This advantage and presence of the contrast between fat and glandular tissues enables sonotomography to clarify the type of glandular tissue. We have confirmed the equal performance of ABVS and MMG in recently published data in detection of the breast type according to BI-RADS ACR type's classification [11]. Thus, ABVS can also be used to evaluate the breast type.

These additional capabilities provided by this method must find their own interpretation in the protocol of examination. Previously during US examination, the gland type and distribution of glandular tissue were hardly described at all; with the development of the automated wide aperture breast sonography, these characteristics should be listed in the protocol. In fatty breast, when no glandular tissue is determined, both breasts are of evenly reduced echogenicity with macrolobulated structure due to the presence of thin fibrous layers between the fat tissues. The

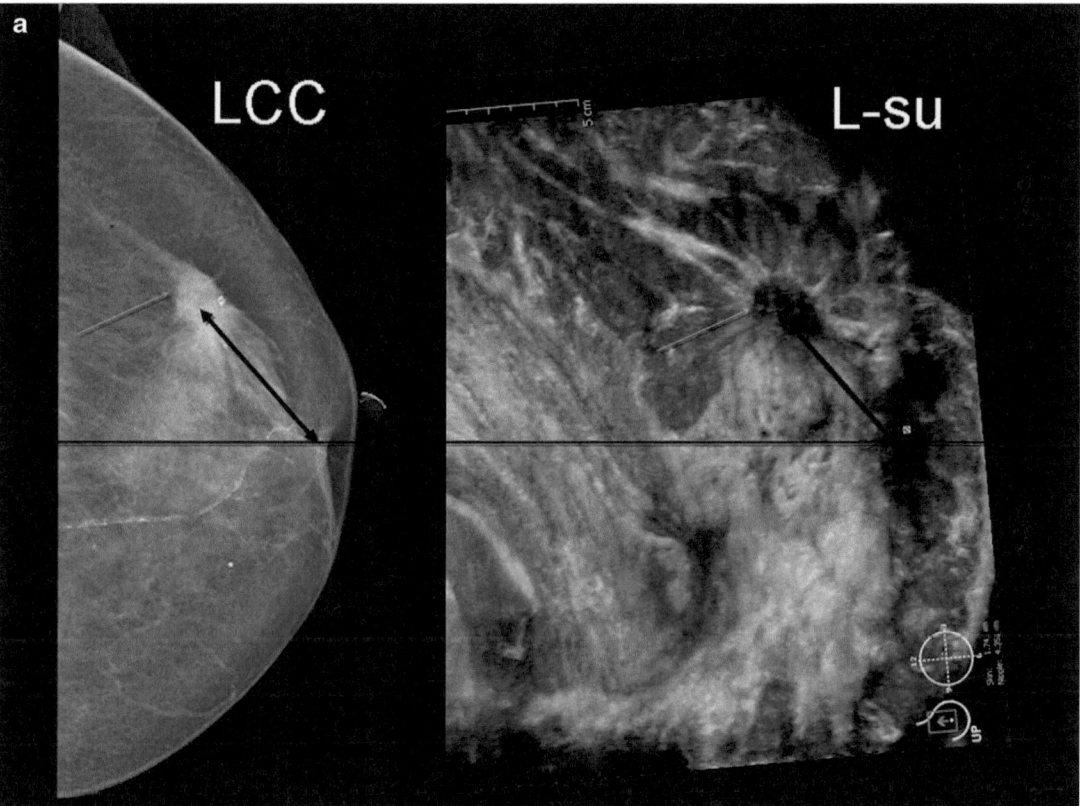

Fig. 3.17 A case of invasive ductal carcinoma in the upper-outer quadrant of the left breast in a 75-year-old woman. Comparison of MMG and ABVS data. Nipple projection is connected by a straight line. (**a**) *Left part*, mammogram in craniocaudal view (L-CC); right part, left superior-to-inferior (L SUP) slice on ABVS (L-SU). The nipple on the MMG is retracted and not seen properly; on the ABVS tomogram, the nipple projection is marked by the *rectangle*. The shadow mass with retraction pattern in the outer quadrant on the MMG coincides with the location of a hypoechoic mass with "spiculated" pattern on the ABVS (*arrows*). The distance from the nipple to the mass is the same in both methods, marked by the thin arrow. (**b**) *Left part*, ABVS tomogram in L MED (mediolateral) view; *right part*, mammogram in mediolateral oblique view—(L-M). The retracted nipple on the MMG is poorly seen; on the ABVS tomogram, the nipple projection is marked by the *rectangle*. The hypoechoic mass in the upper quadrant of the left gland on the ABVS image coincides with the shadow streaking mass on the MMG. The distance from the nipple to the mass is comparable in both methods and marked by a *thin arrow*

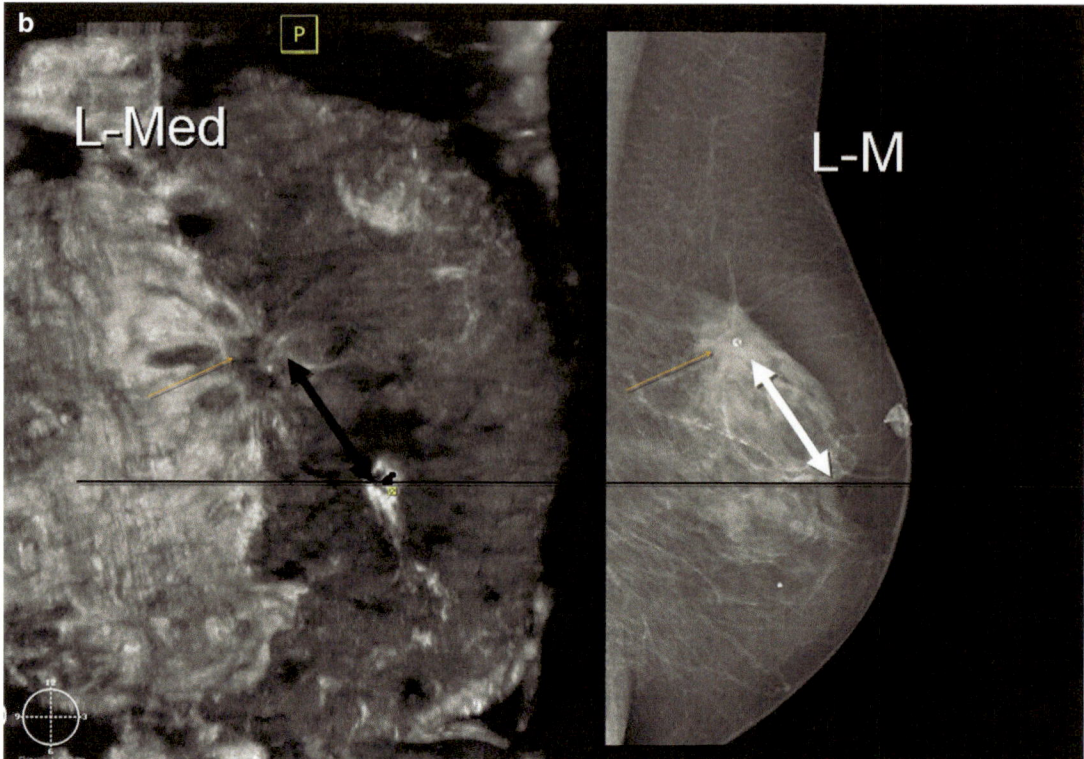

Fig. 3.17 (continued)

ABVS structure of the adipose involution of the breast coincides fully with the MMG image (Fig. 3.22). When the residual glandular tissue is located predominantly in the upper-outer quadrants, its topography can also be documented using ABVS tomography (Fig. 3.23). The diagnosis of breast pathology in women with glandular-type ACR III and ACR IV BI-RADS breasts by mammography is difficult. Therefore, in these cases, the examination should include US study or ABVS tomography examination (Figs. 3.24 and 3.25). In hyperechoic fibroglandular tissue, any hypoechoic breast masses are identified easier and better with ultrasonography. The only exception is microcalcifications which are a particular use case for US.

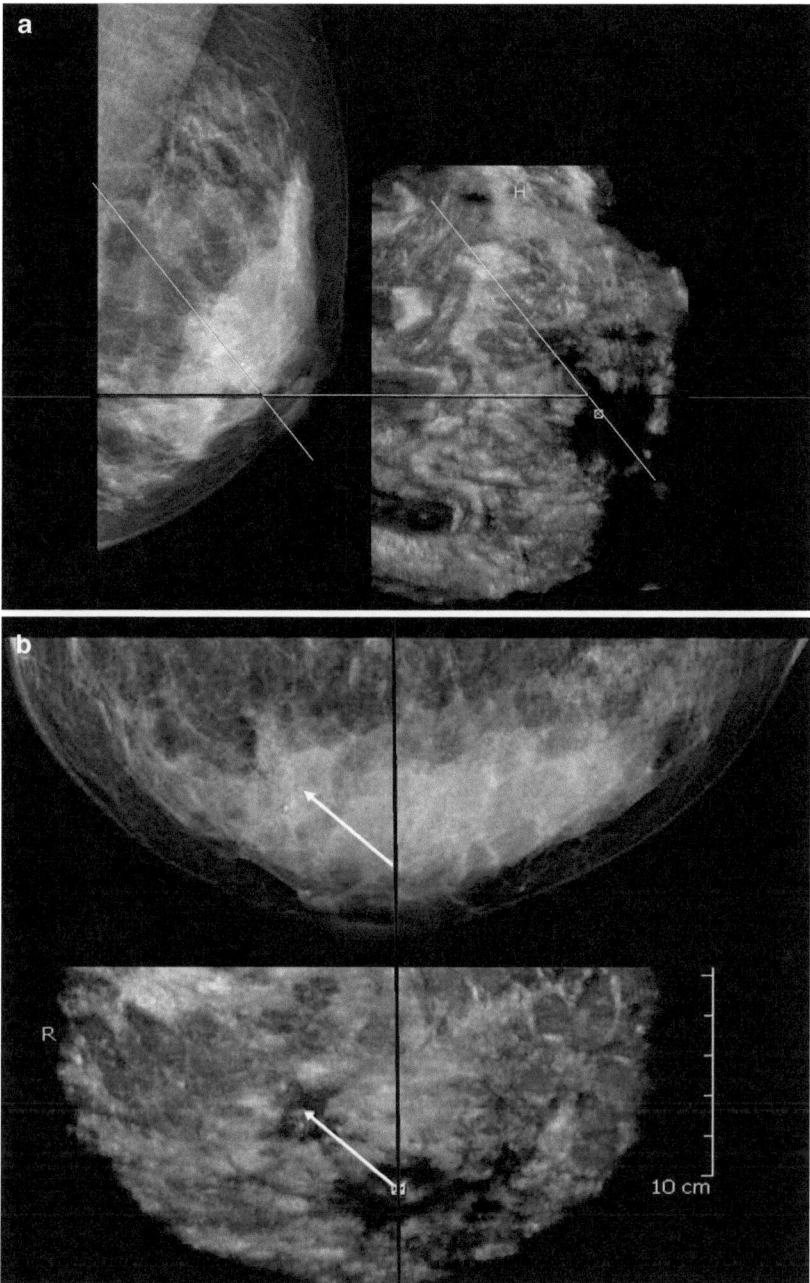

Fig. 3.18 A case of invasive ductal carcinoma in the upper-internal quadrant of the left breast in a 38-year-old woman. Comparison of MMG and ABVS data. Detection of the lesion in dense breast found by ABVS by mapping it on the MMG. The nipple line is marked by a straight line. Note the distance between the nipple and the lesion is equal on both images. (**a**) *Left part*, mammogram in mediolateral oblique view; *right part*, ABVS tomogram in latero-medial view. The tumor on the MMG is present as a zone of focal microcalcification against the dense glandular tissue. The tumor and the nipple are connected with a continuing direct (*white*) line. ABVS shows a hypoechoic area with irregular stellate margins in this view. The distance from the nipple to the mass is comparable in both methods. (**b**) *On the top*, mammogram in craniocaudal view; *on the bottom*, superior-to-inferior slice on ABVS. Hypoechoic mass with irregular contours is clearly visible on the ABVS image (*white arrow*). It matches the grouped microcalcifications on the dense glandular tissue on the MMG (*arrow*). The distance from the nipple to the mass is the same in both methods

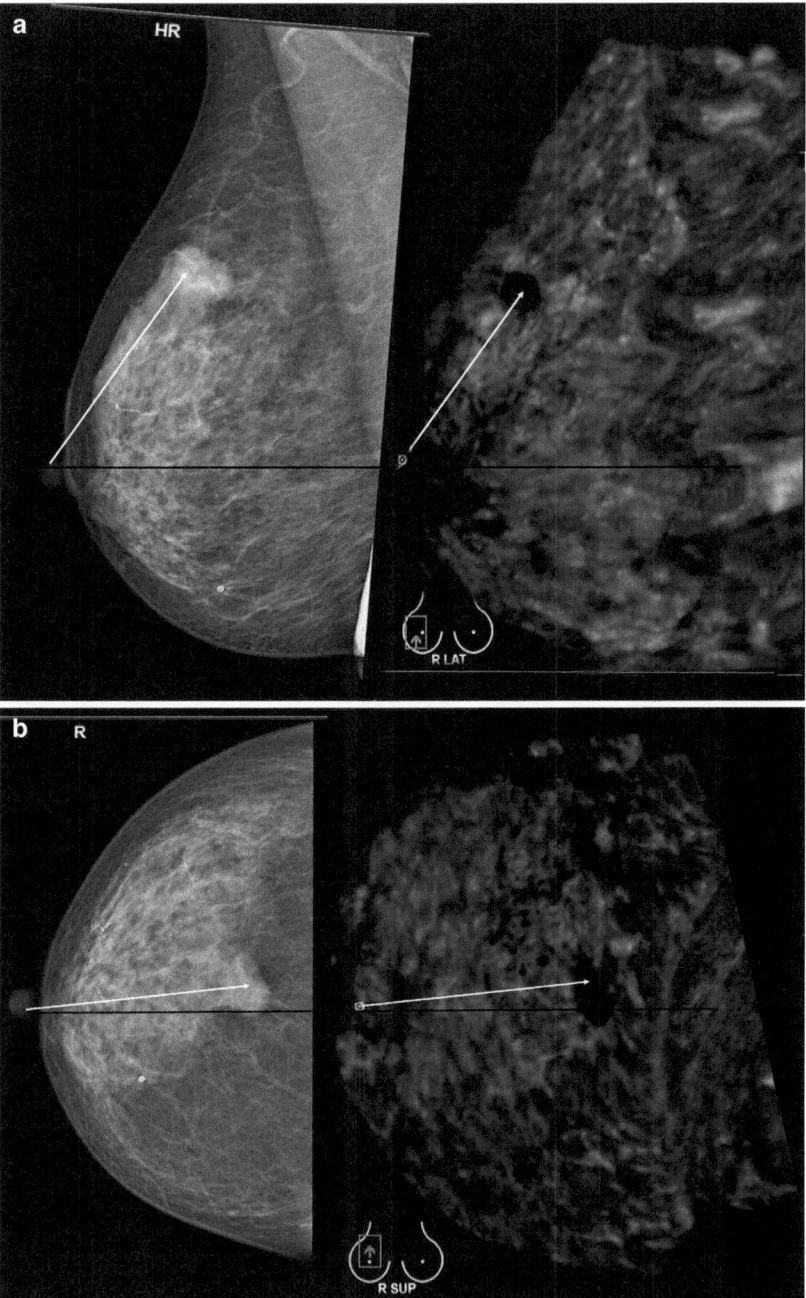

Fig. 3.19 A case of invasive ductal carcinoma in the middle of the upper quadrants of the right breast in a 62-year-old woman. Comparison of MMG and ABVS data. Nipple line is marked by a straight line (*black line*). The tumor and the nipple are connected by the line. (**a**) *Left part*, mammogram in mediolateral oblique view; right part, ABVS tomogram in latero-medial view. MMG shows a hyperdense round mass with a slight retraction pattern, which corresponds to the hypoechoic nodule on the ABVS tomo-gram with a hyperechoic irregular thick rim. The distance from the nipple to the mass is the same in both methods (*white arrow*). (**b**) *Left part*, mammogram in craniocaudal view; *right part*, right superior-to-inferior (R SUP) slice on ABVS. Centrally positioned dense nodule in the deep part of the breast on the MMG corresponds to the hypoechoic oval-shaped nodule with slight spiculated boundaries on the ABVS tomogram. The same distance from the nipple to the mass in both methods (*white arrow*)

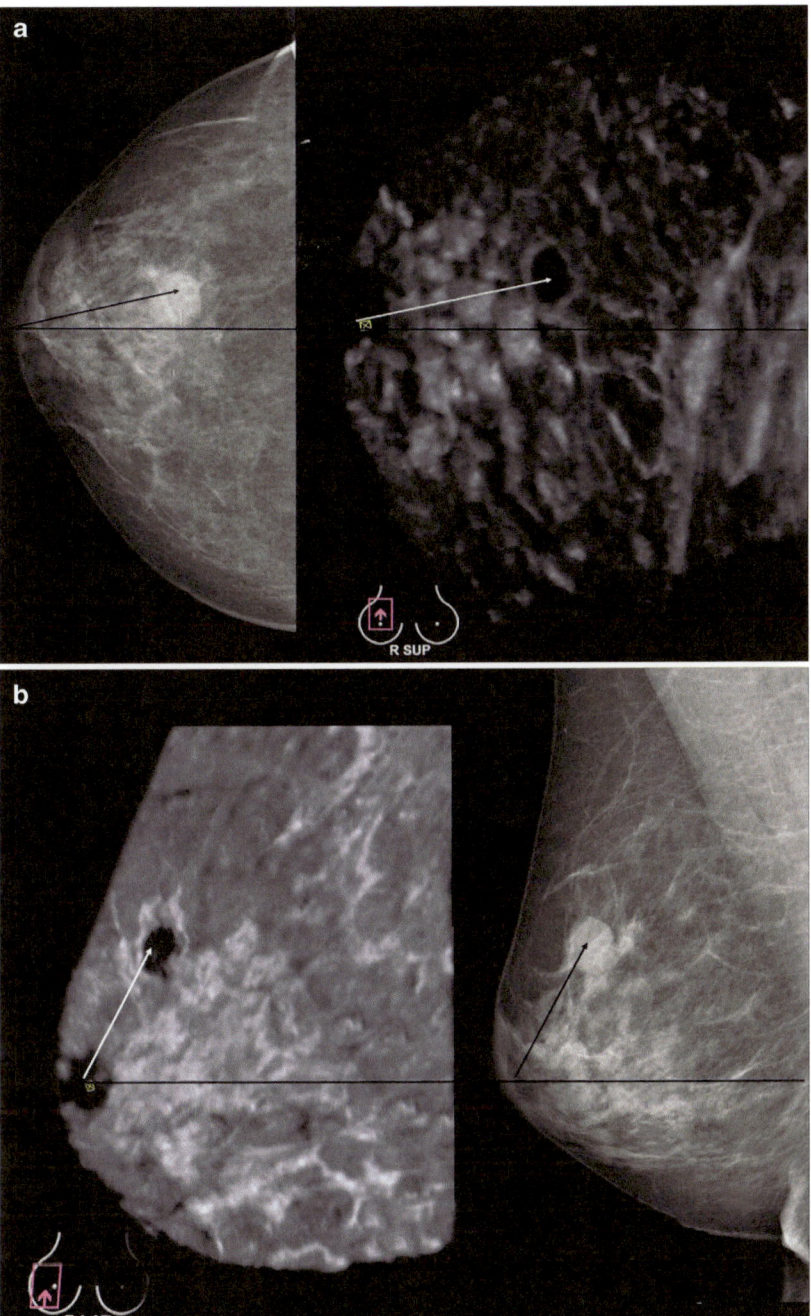

Fig. 3.20 A case of intracanalicular fibroadenomas in the upper-outer quadrant of the right breast. A comparison between MMG and ABVS data. Nipple line is marked by a straight line (*black line*). Identification of the lesions in the radiodense breast with ABVS and their projection on MMG. An equal distance from the nipple to the lesion is seen on both images. (**a**) *Left part*, R SUP (right superior-to-inferior) slice on ABVS; *right part*, mammogram in craniocaudal view. Dense nodule in the deep part of the outer breast on the MMG corresponds to the hypoechoic oval-shaped nodule with a clear thin round rim. Note the equal distance between the nipple and the nodule shown by both methods. (**b**) *Left part*, ABVS tomogram in R LAT (latero-medial) view; *right part*, mammogram in mediolateral oblique view. Hypoechoic nodule with hyperechoic thin rim with regular margins is clearly seen in the upper quadrant on the ABVS tomogram (*white arrow*) which corresponds to the oval-shaped dense nodule with clear margins and compression phenomenon on the MMG (*black arrow*)

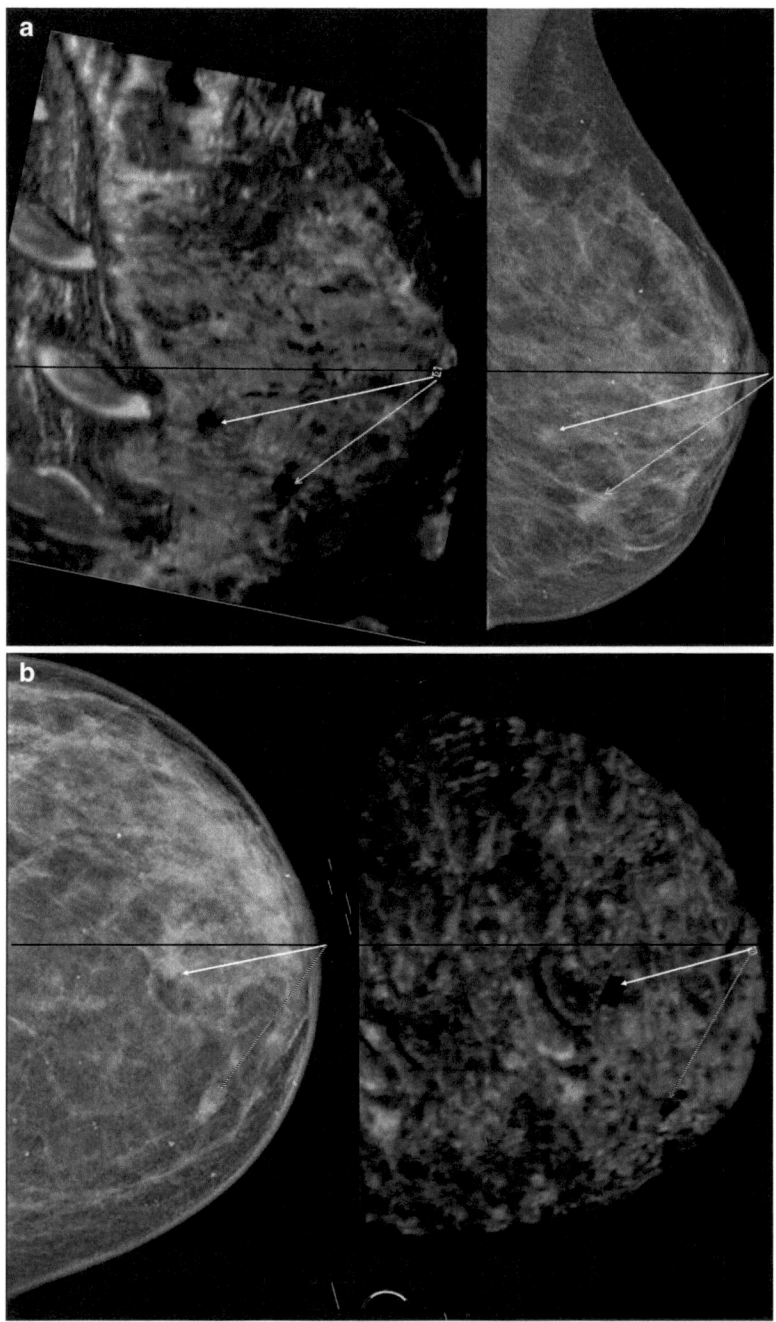

Fig. 3.21 A case of multifocal invasive lobular carcinoma of the lower-inner quadrant of the left breast in a 49-year-old female patient. The significant breast density identified as ACR IV-type BI-RADS classification. Comparison of MMG and ABVS data. The black line goes through the nipples. (**a**) *Left part*, ABVS tomogram in L MED (mediolateral) view; *right part*, mammogram in mediolateral oblique view. The mammogram reveals two subtle isodense nodules with blurred contours and without a strong desmoplastic response (*two white arrows*), which were assessed as multifocal malignancies. The ABVS found two subtle hypoechoic lesions clearly visible through the echogenic glandular tissue with a slight radiant pattern and irregular contours (*two white arrows*). (**b**) *Left part*, mammogram in craniocaudal view; *right part*, left superior-to-inferior slice on ABVS. The two lesions of polygonal shape with a slight radiance are clearly visible on the ABVS tomogram. The projection of the masses from the ABVS on the mammogram helps to clarify the localization of the second lesion, undetermined on the CC view due to its overlapping by radiodense breast tissue, and helps to confirm the multifocality of the process

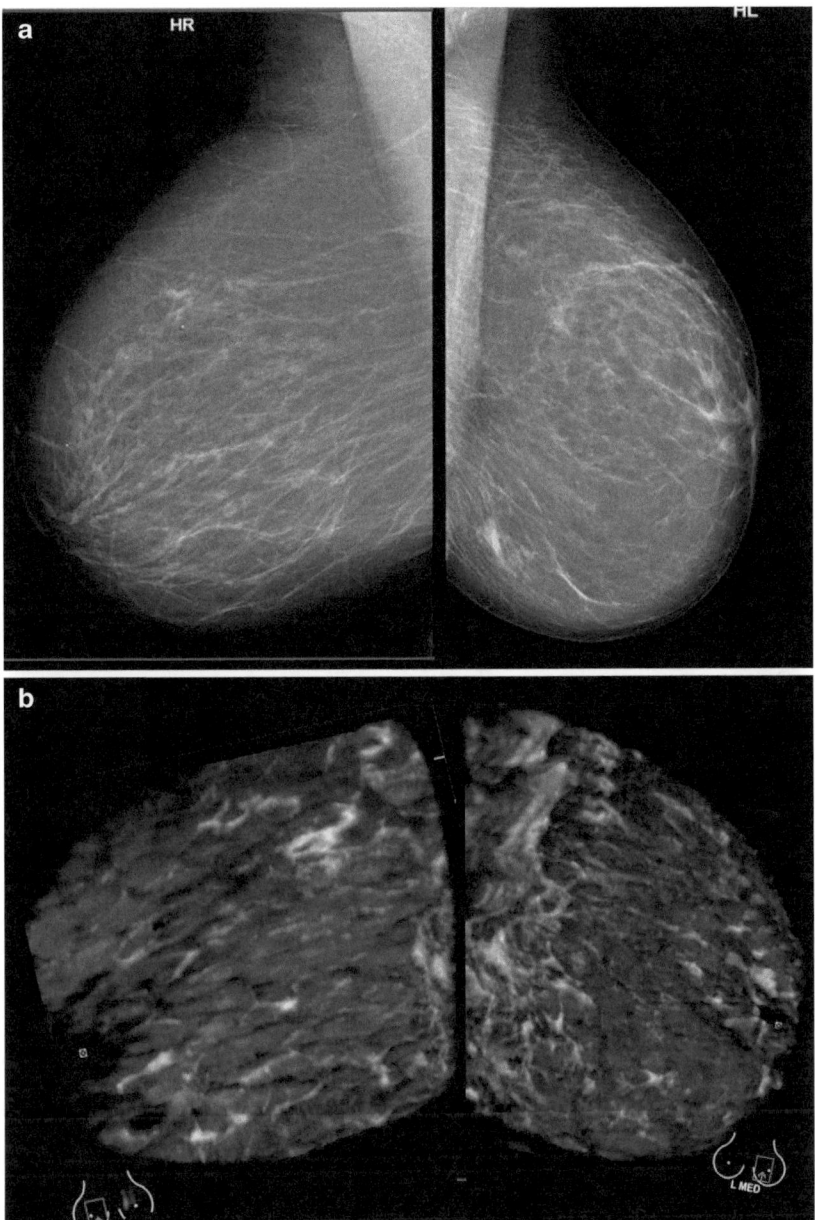

Fig. 3.22 A case demonstration of the ACR I fatty breast type in a 68-year-old woman. Comparison of MMG and ABVS data. Marked asymmetry of breast development is visible and identified by both methods with the same proportions. (**a**) A side-by-side mammography of the breasts. Oblique mediolateral views of both glands showed the marked prevalence of the right breast size. (**b**) Oblique mediolateral ABVS side-by-side tomograms of both glands in similar projections rotated to compare with the mammograms. The asymmetry is also defined on the ABVS

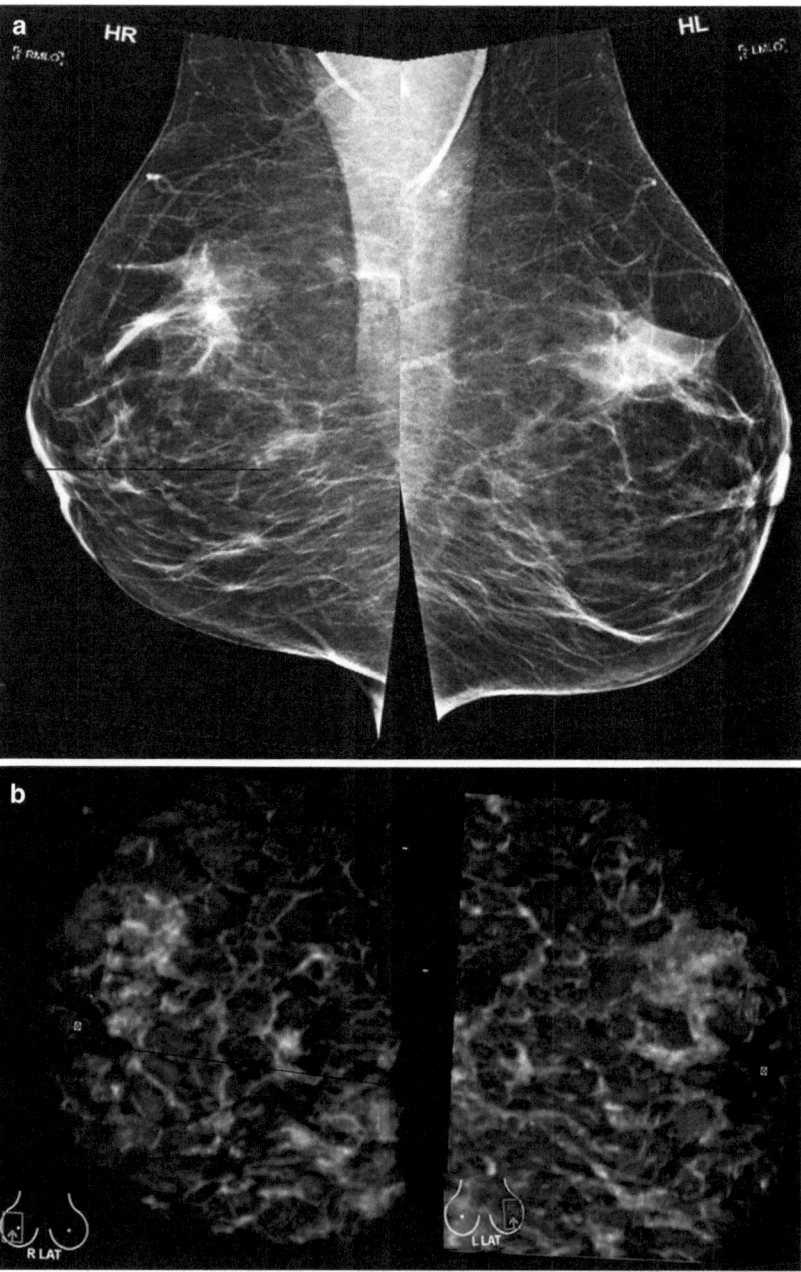

Fig. 3.23 A case demonstration of the ACR II-type breast with residual glandular tissue presented in the upper quadrants in a 55-year-old female patient. Comparison of both breasts on MMG and SABVS images. (**a**) Side-by-side mammography of the breasts. Oblique mediolateral views of both glands show a low amount of radiolucent tissue in the upper quadrants. (**b**) Oblique latero-medial ABVS side-by-side tomograms of both glands in similar projections demonstrate hyperechoic areas which correspond to the glandular tissue. The distribution is quite similar to those on the MMG

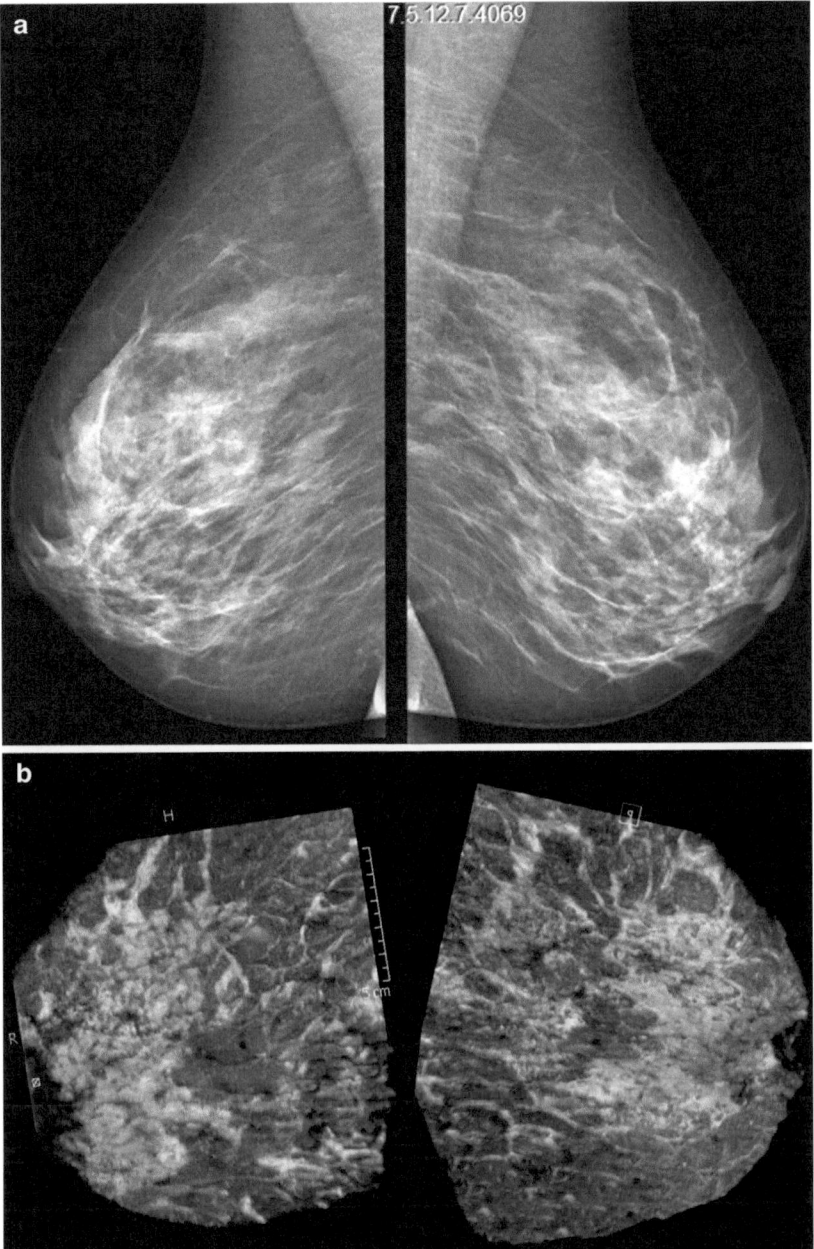

Fig. 3.24 A case of ACR III breast type with benign fibrocystic disease in a 51-year-old woman with hormone replacement therapy. Comparison of MMG and ABVS data. The residual glandular tissue—more than 50 % but less than 75 %. (**a**) Side-by-side mammography of the breasts. Oblique mediolateral views of both glands show an increase in the amount of glandular tissue with fibrous component in both breasts. (**b**) Oblique latero-medial ABVS side-by-side tomograms of both glands in similar projections demonstrate hyperechoic fibroglandular tissue with an amount of more than 50 % in both glands. The tissue structure is quite similar to those on the MMG

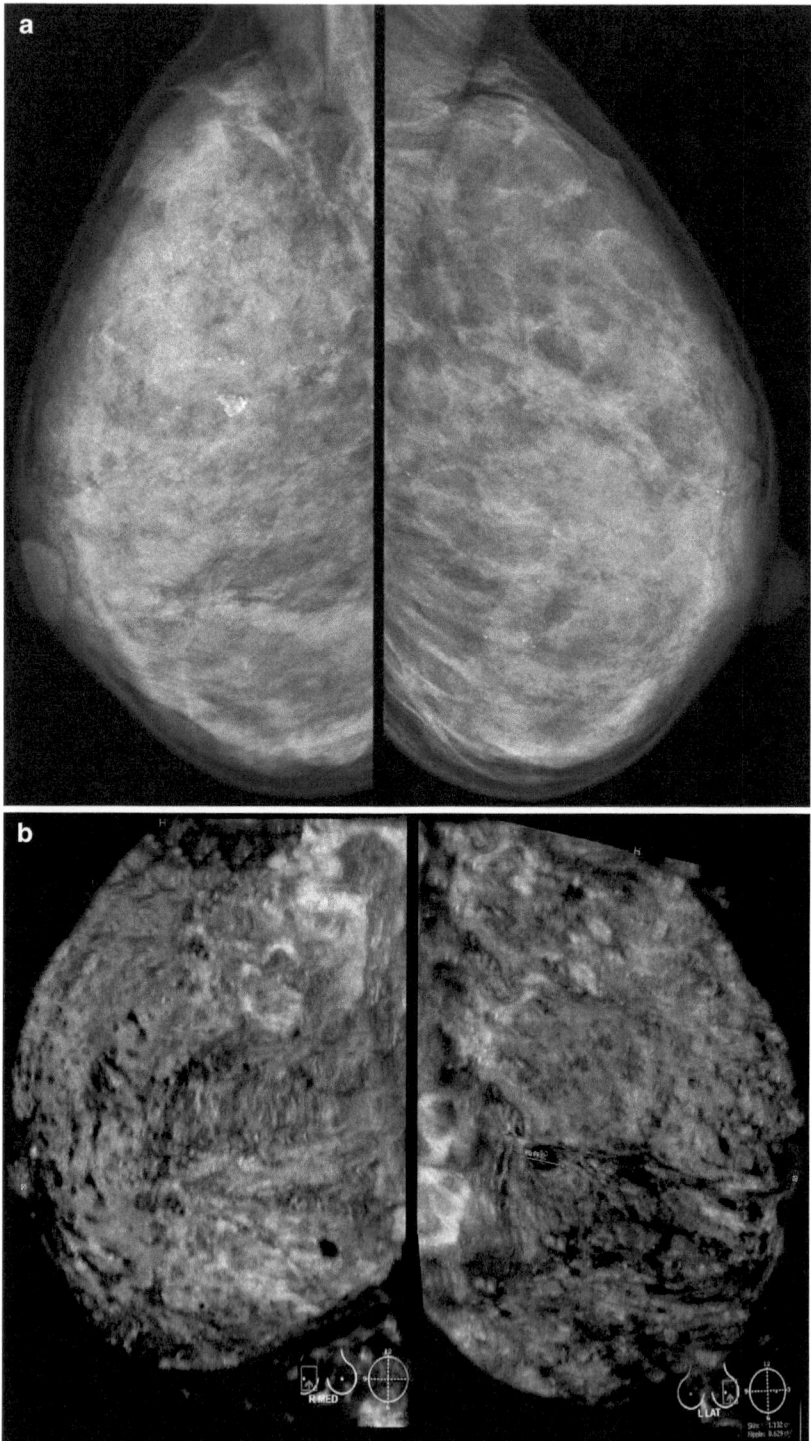

Fig. 3.25 A case of the ACR IV breast type according to BI-RADS. Significantly dense breast in all regions in a female patient of 55 with diabetes mellitus. Comparison of both breasts on MMG and ABVS images. (**a**) Side-by-side mammography of the breasts. Oblique mediolateral views of both glands. The absence of pre- and retromammary fat tissue, compression of the breasts with slight deformity due to severe fibrous changes. (**b**) Oblique latero-medial ABVS side-by-side tomograms of both glands in similar projections. The whole gland shows glandular and fibrous tissue with the same absence of fatty zone in the retromammary space

Literature

1. Lindenbraten LD, Burdina LM, Pinhosevich YeG (1997) Mammography (Educational Atlas): M. LLP "Vidar" (book in Russian)
2. Sickles EA (1997) Management of lesions appearing probably benign at mammography. In: Friedrich M, Sickles EA (eds) Radiological diagnosis of breast diseases. Springer, Berlin/Heidelberg/New York, pp 167–172
3. Stavros AT, Thickmann D, Rapp CL et al (1995) Solid breast nodules: use of sonography to determine between benign and malignant nodules. Radiology 196:123–134
4. Boyd NF, Guo H, Martin LJ et al (2007) Mammographic density and the risk and detection of breast cancer. N Engl J Med 356:227–236
5. Buist DS, Porter PL, Lehman C et al (2004) Factors contributing to mammography failure in women aged 40–49 years. J Natl Cancer Inst 96:1432–1440
6. Carney PA, Miglioretti DL, Yankaskas BC et al (2003) Individual and combined effects of age, breast density, and hormone replacement therapy use on the accuracy of screening mammography. Ann Intern Med 138:168–175
7. Hooley RJ, Greenberg KL, Stackhouse RM et al (2012) Screening US in patients with mammographically dense breasts: initial experience with Connecticut Public Act 09–41. Radiology 265:59–69
8. Kelly KM, Dean J, Comulada WS et al (2010) Breast cancer detection using automated whole breast ultrasound and mammography in radiographically dense breasts. Eur Radiol 20:734–742
9. Duric N, Boyd N, Littrup P et al (2013) Breast density measurements with ultrasound tomography: a comparison with film and digital mammography. Med Phys 40(1):013501–013512
10. Sak M (2011) Relationship between breast sound speed and mammographic percent density. Proc. SPIE7968, Medical Imaging: Ultrasonic Imaging, Tomography, and Therapy, 79680N (March 25, 2011)
11. Gazhonova VE, Efremova MP, Bachurina EM et al (2015) The possibilities of assessing the glandular type of the breast structure by sonotomography from the standpoint of the risk factor for breast cancer development. Ann Roentgenol Radiol 5:23–29 (article in Russian)

4.1 Normal Breast

Currently MMG is accepted as a "gold standard" in the evaluation of breast diseases in patients older than 40. The ultrasound technique is widely used in young women for examination of the breast structure. ABVS opens a new approach to assessment of breast anatomy, with visualization of the whole gland at once allowing analysis of all observed changes in relation to other X-ray and MR modalities and good reproducibility of the corresponding images during follow-up.

Normal breast structure varies over time in the same women, during the menstrual cycle, pregnancy, after weaning, and during menopause [1–3]. This variability is also reflected in the ABVS images.

The female breast is composed of glandular, fatty tissue interspersed with fibrous or connective tissue. The distribution and prevalence of the fatty or glandular tissue depends on age and hormonal changes [4–8]. Thick fascia covering the pectoralis major and serratus anterior muscles make up the bed of the breast. Layers of premammary superficial and retromammary deep fatty tissue surround the gland. Chest and intercostal muscles are located posterior to the pectoral fascia. Fibrous septa extend from the dermis into the breast parenchyma to create the Cooper suspensory ligaments. They divide the gland into 15–25 cone-shaped functional lobes which are distributed in the fibrofatty stroma in multiple lobules. The lobes are arranged radially around the nipple with apices turned to it. The lobes drain into multiple ducts which coalesce and subsequently drain into lactiferous ducts which terminate at the nipple. The breast lobule consists of 20–40 acini or alveoli which are the main secretory unit of the breast tissue. The lobule and the first terminal duct arising from it constitute the terminal ductlobular unit (TDLU). The TDLU is an important site for the development of cancer and benign proliferations of the breast [1].

The breast fibroglandular stroma is a clinically important structure consisting of supporting stroma and periglandular stroma. The supporting stroma is formed from processes of the superficial fascia and interlobular layers consisting of coarse connective tissue from collagen fibers, relatively poor in cells. The periglandular stroma immediately surrounds the ducts and has a loose soft fibrous structure, with abundant fibroblasts and several macrophages, lymphocytes, and plasma cells. The expression of the periglandular stroma is proportional to the development of the glandular tissue. The supporting stroma and periglandular stroma absorb X-rays equally and therefore they cannot be differentiated mammographically, appearing as continuous glandular tissue. The mammographic density of the breast depends on the amount of these stromal and epithelial elements. Increased MMG density is more apparent in young women than postmenopausal women.

In young women, the differences between supporting and periglandular stromata can be

V. Gazhonova, *3D Automated Breast Volume Sonography*, DOI 10.1007/978-3-319-41971-8_4

seen with the help of ultrasound. The supporting stroma appears on sonograms as areas of increased echogenicity. On the contrary, periglandular stroma is seen as low echogenicity areas. These two structures should be considered as glandular tissue during ultrasound imaging analysis to enable comparisons between MMG and US. Thus, breasts in the early reproductive period (at the age of 15–25) have a cellular structure with alternating zones of low and high echogenicity. This variability of the echostructure is provided by the periglandular stroma. The structure of the glandular tissue varies from reticular to cellular in young women with a regular menstrual cycle. Edema and hyperemia of the periglandular stroma decrease echogenicity and provide a reticular pattern in the secretory phase. The periglandular stroma narrows, and the echogenicity of the glandular tissue increases with less expressed nodularity in the proliferation phase. The echostructure becomes cellular. The additional hypoechoic masses are identified more easily against this background in the proliferation phase (Figs. 4.1 and 4.2). Therefore, the

proliferative phase of the menstrual cycle also is preferable for examining the breast with 3DUS in the reproductive period, as in conventional 2D ultrasound. Collapsed ducts are not clearly visible in the proliferative phase against a background of echogenic glandular tissue. They can sometimes be seen in the secretory phase of MC as hyperechoic dots or lines.

Glandular tissue occupies practically all areas of the gland in the early reproductive period and can be clearly seen in the anterior and posterior slices of a full-sized image (Fig. 4.3). Adipose tissue is expressed minimally. Cooper's ligaments cannot be clearly visualized on the background of this high echogenic glandular tissue. The nipple is represented as a hyperechoic ovoid structure with a minimal hypoechoic distal shadow.

The structure of the right and left breasts is basically quite symmetrical. If any asymmetry is present, pathology should be excluded [3]. This was stated in relation to MMG but can be applied to ABVS as well. Computer workstations allow assessing the right and left breast by matching

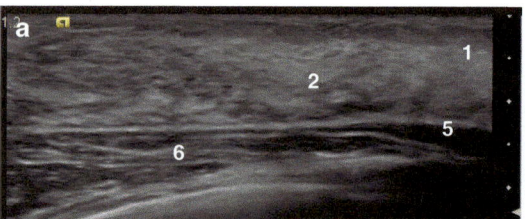
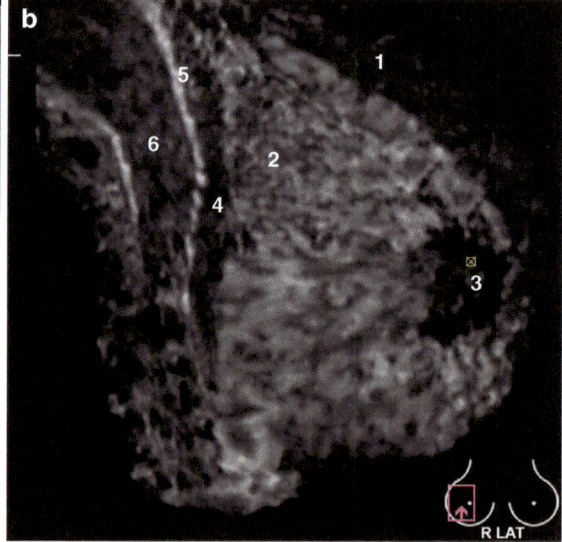

Fig. 4.1 A case of normal breast in a 20-year-old woman, without a history of pregnancy. Proliferation phase. Hyperechoic glandular tissue. Cellular pattern of breast structure due to the balanced development of supporting and periglandular stroma. (1) Premammary fat, (2) glandular tissue, (3) nipple and areolar area, (4) retromammary fat, (5) superficial fascia, (6) pectoral muscles.

Comparison of data of the same patient in conventional 2D HHUS and ABVS images. (**a**) HHUS image with a small field of view depicting part of the gland, (**b**) ABVS tomogram in R LAT (latero-medial) view of the right breast. The rectangle marks the nipple area. ABVS showed close to "anatomical" visualization of the breast structures

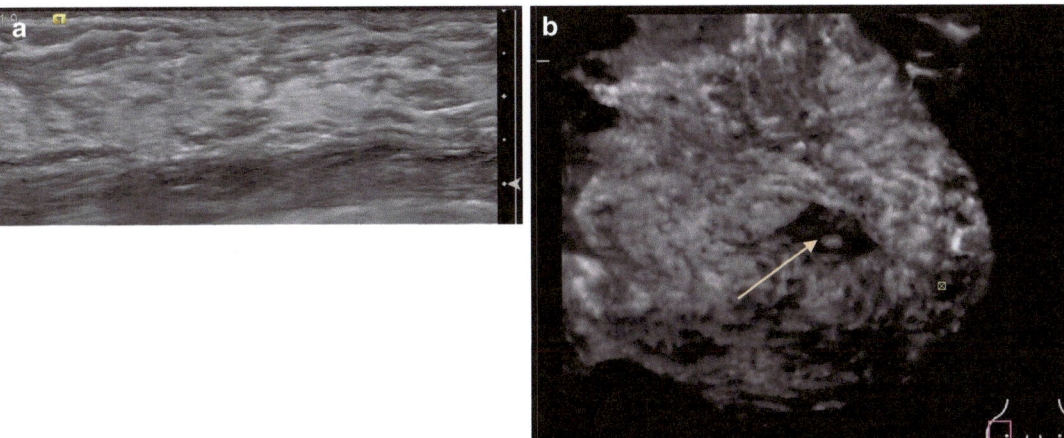

Fig. 4.2 Breast in the proliferation phase of the menstrual cycle in a 30-year-old woman without a history of a pregnancy. Note the good contrast between the glandular tissue and the lesion (fibroadenoma). Comparison of data for the same patient in conventional 2D HHUS and ABVS images. (**a**) HHUS image depicting the glandular tissue in a line-structure pattern. (**b**) ABVS tomogram in R LAT (latero-medial) view of the right breast. Hypoechogenic fibroadenoma (*arrow*) in the upper part of the breast is clearly visible against the background of highly echogenic glandular tissue which is more prominent than the fatty tissue. *Rectangle marks* the nipple

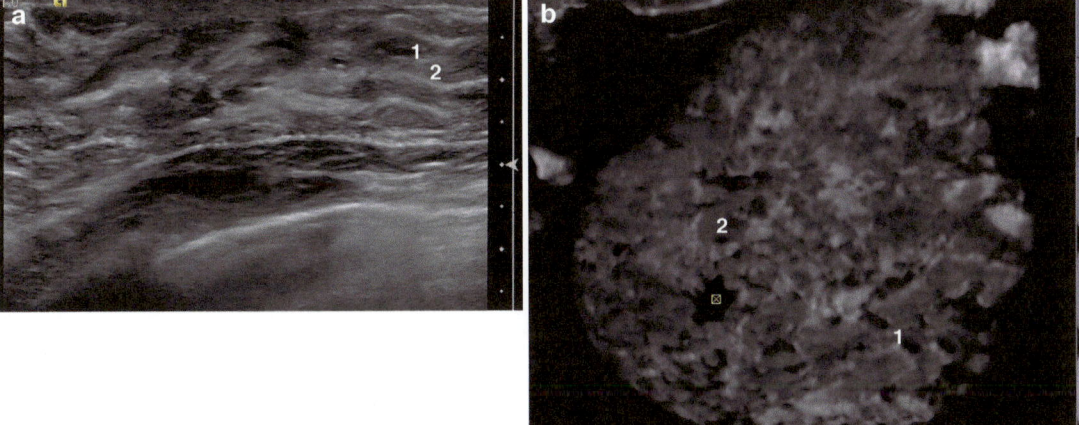

Fig. 4.3 Breast in the secretory phase of the menstrual cycle in a 28-year-old woman, nulliparous. Thickened hypoechoic periglandular stroma (2). The anechoic structure inside the stroma corresponds to the slightly dilated ducts (1) in the secretory phase of the menstrual cycle. Comparison of data of the same patient in conventional 2D HHUS and ABVS images. (**a**) HHUS image depicts thickened glandular tissue and a decrease in echogenicity of the breast with ill-defined line-structures. (**b**) ABVS tomogram of the left breast. *L AP*—left anteroposterior coronal slice. Uniform decrease of echogenicity of the breast parenchyma. Small anechoic areas correspond to enlarged ducts

slices. These images and saved clips from the whole array of ultrasound data facilitate identification of developmental abnormalities, the preferential location of the glandular tissue, its distribution per quadrants, its structural features, and pathological masses (Fig. 4.4). The adaptive mode offered by ABVS—nipple shadow reduction tool—improves visualization of the retroareolar structures. 3D data should be acquired using the nipple maximum lateralization technique; it helps to reduce the "no-show" areas under the nipple and retroareolar region on LAT (latero-medial oblique) and SUP (superior craniocaudal) views. With a conventional 2D US technique, the visualization of retroareolar regions without informational and quality loss usually requires the additional use of a water paddle.

The most intensive breast development starts at the end of pregnancy and in lactation. During pregnancy, the breasts are influenced by hor-mones produced by the placenta, with hyperpla-sia of glandular lobes and increase development of ducts. At the end of pregnancy, the breast loses the cellular structure and appears as a uniform thickened layer of glandular tissue. In this period, TDLU transform and develop fur-ther, connective tissue septa are stretched and thinned, and edema and increased vascularity are present. Echogenic layers of supporting stroma are correspondingly thin on a sonogram. ABVS shows these changes as a loss of reticular struc-ture, even a decrease in echogenicity of the glan-dular tissue, with several subtle hyperechoic linear structures (ducts), mainly in areolar areas (Fig. 4.5). After lactation, the breast lobules involute following the withdrawal of prolactin stimulation. On ABVS, cellular or reticular breast structure is restored.

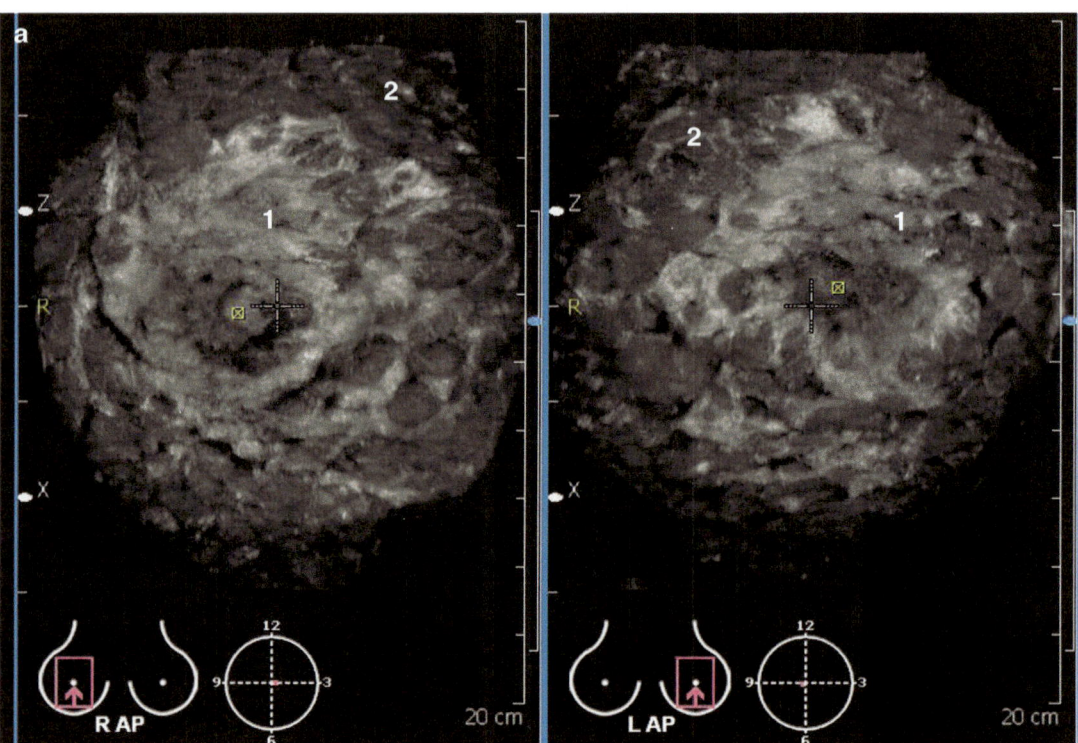

Fig. 4.4 Analysis of the breast structure using ABVS data on a workstation and US device. (**a**) ABVS worksta-tion side-by-side comparison of the right (*left part of pic-ture*) and the left (*right part of picture*) breast in coronal anteroposterior views at the level of the glandular triangle (20 mm in depth from the nipple). The type of view is indicated by the icon. The nipple is marked in the center of each breast by a *rectangle*. The structure of both breasts is symmetrical lobulated with a medium amount of fatty tissue. Glandular tissue is distributed around the nipple equally. The region under the nipple is seen with-out "no-show" zones. (**b**) ABVS multislice mode analysis on a US device. R MED view (mediolateral oblique view) of the right breast. The depth of each slice is marked from 75 to 84 mm from the medial part to the lateral part. Fifty-six slices were obtained with a slice thickness of 3 mm. These four images (25/56, 26/56, 27/56, 28/56 slices) were selected to show the structure of the middle part of the breast, and they could be com-pared with corresponding slices in digital breast tomo-synthesis. The nipple is marked by a rectangle. Note a hypoechoic area in the retroareolar region. Slight cellu-larity of the glandular tissue corresponds to the early reproductive type of the breast

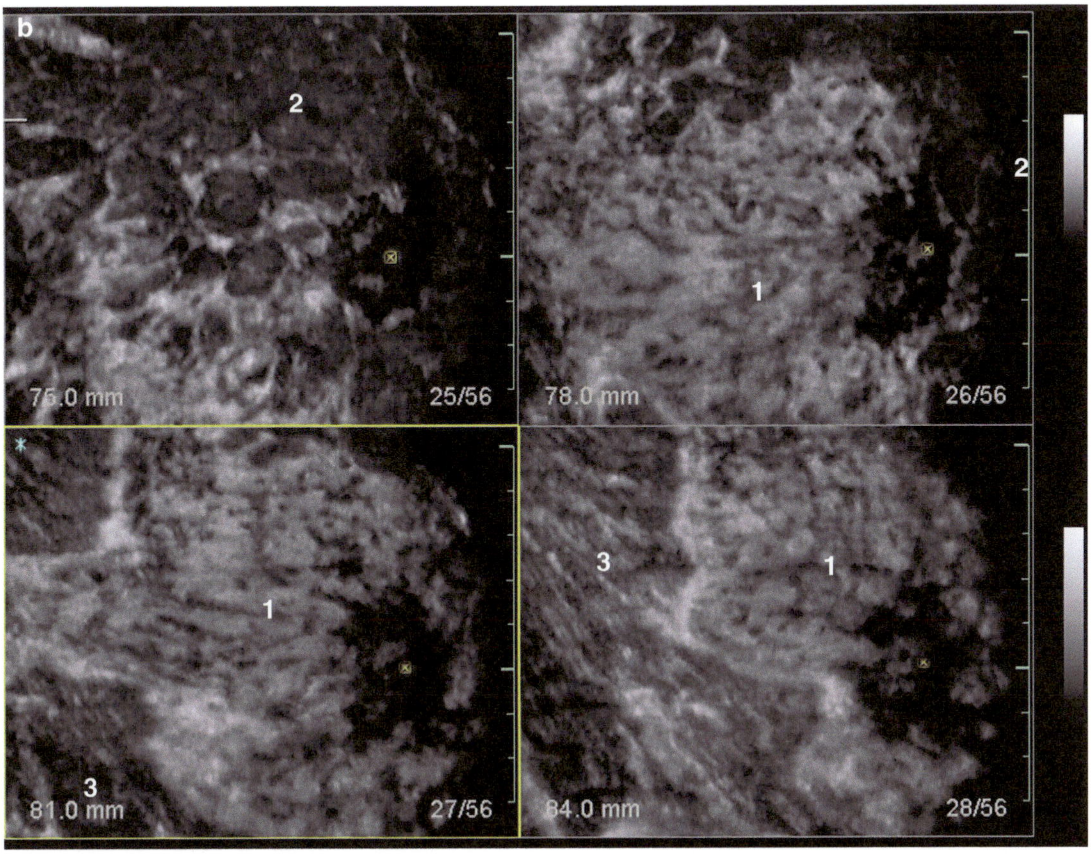

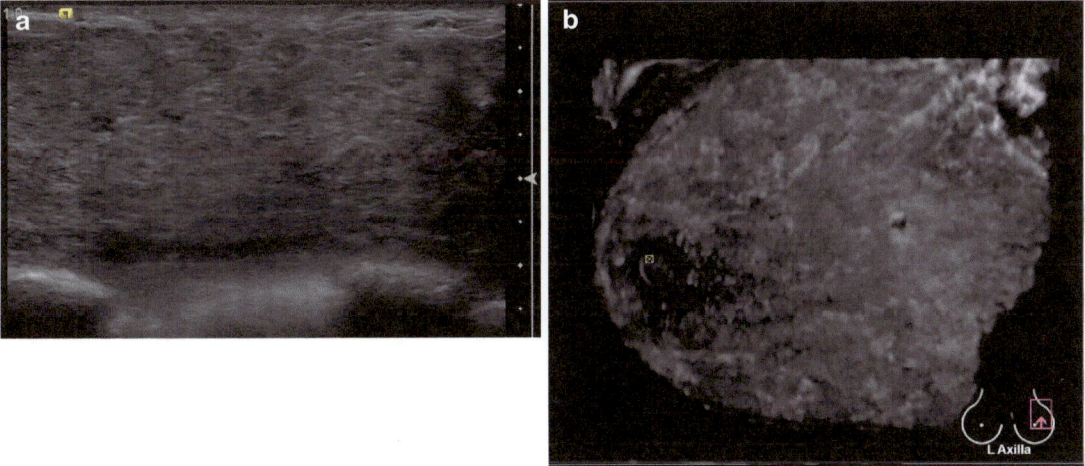

Fig. 4.4 (continued)

Fig. 4.5 Breast during lactation. Comparison of data for the same patient in conventional 2D HHUS and ABVS images. (**a**) On an HHUS image, the absence of pre- and retromammary fat tissue is noted. An absence of cellularity, a uniform decrease in echogenicity of the glandular tissue. The absence of interlobular fat and fibrous tissue. Linear horizontal stripes indicate the milk ducts. (**b**) ABVS image from L-axilla view (axillary oblique view of the left breast). The breast consists only of glandular tissue of low echogenicity. Note the homogeneity of the breast parenchyma during lactation

At the age of 35 or sometimes earlier, fat tissue appears in between the glandular tissues, even in lean-bodied women. Areas of the breast between the fat lobes mostly still have a cellular structure. Later, at the age of 40, the proportion of fatty tissue is further increased, and the glandular tissue loses its cellular pattern due to interlobular fibrosis (Figs. 4.6, 4.7, and 4.8).

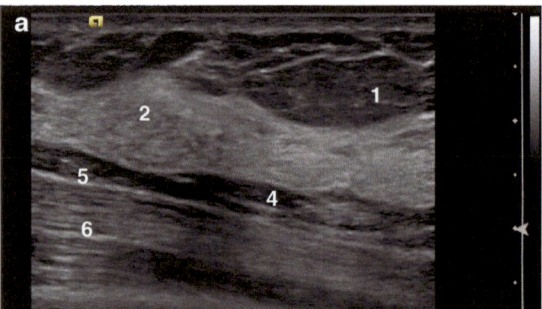
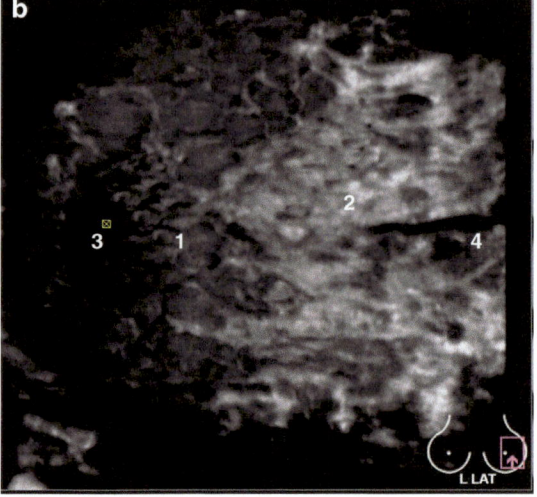

Fig. 4.6 Breast structure in the late reproductive period in a 36-year-old woman 1 year after pregnancy and lactation. Comparison of data for the same patient in conventional 2D HHUS and ABVS images. (1) Premammary fat, (2) glandular tissue, (3) nipple and areolar area, (4) retromammary fat, (5) superficial fascia, (6) pectoral muscles. (**a**) HHUS image shows disappearance of cellularity of the breast tissue and increase in echogenicity due to involution process in the stroma. Enlargement of pre- and retromammary spaces. (**b**) ABVS tomogram of the left breast obtained in the LAT view (left latero-medial oblique view). Increased echogenicity of the breast tissue and prominent fatty tissue in the premammary region

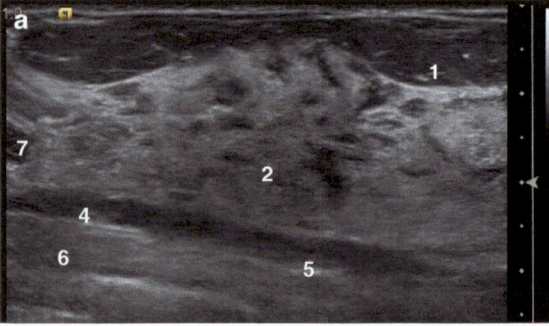
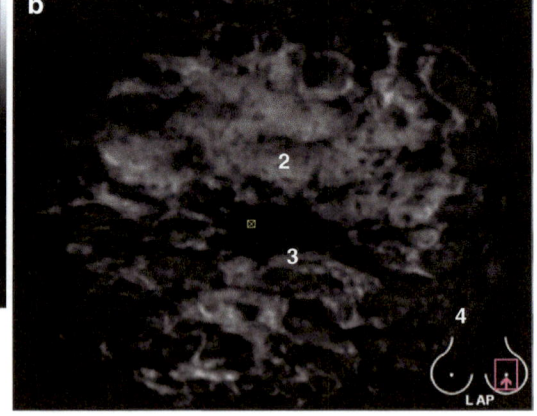

Fig. 4.7 Breast structure in the late reproductive period in a 45-year-old female without a history of lactation. Comparison of conventional 2D HHUS and ABVS images of the same patient. Key: (1) premammary fat, (2) glandular tissue, (3) nipple and areolar area, (4) retromammary fat, (5) superficial fascia, (6) pectoral muscles, (7) Cooper's ligaments. (**a**) On HHUS image stroma is echogenic with areas of preserved cellularity. Premammary fat space is more prominent than in the early reproductive period. (**b**) ABVS tomogram of the left breast obtained in the AP view (coronal anteroposterior view). The distribution of glandular tissue is located mainly in the upper quadrants, with fatty tissue dominating in the lower quadrants

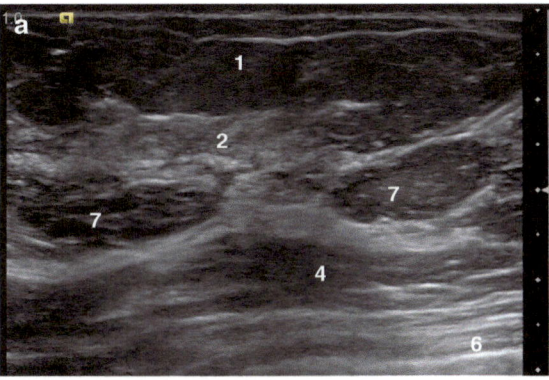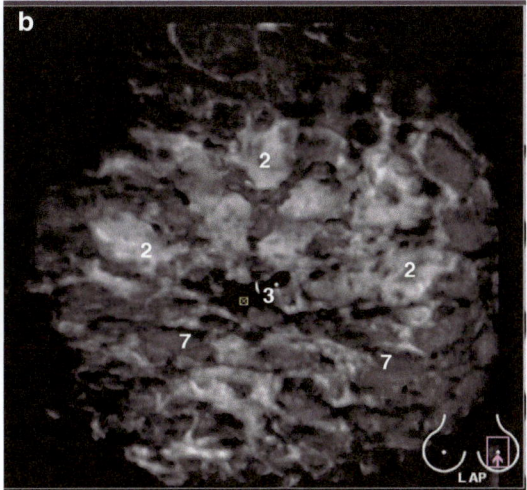

Fig. 4.8 Involution changes of the breast in a premenopausal 48-year-old woman. Comparison of the HHUS and ABVS data of the same patient. (1) Premammary fat, (2) glandular tissue, (3) nipple and areolar area, (4) retromammary fat, (6) pectoral muscles, (7) Cooper's ligaments. (**a**) On the HHUS image reduction and narrowing of the echogenic glandular tissue, increase of fibrosis and appearance of fatty lobes interspersed in the residual glandular tissue are clearly seen. (**b**) ABVS tomogram of the left breast obtained in AP view (coronal anteroposterior view). **1** The whole-breast structure is shown with a distribution pattern of echogenic glandular lobes interrupted by fatty lobules. Thin strip lines of residual stroma are seen as hyperechoic lines

At the age of 50–60, the proportion of fatty tissue in the breast increases even more. The breast tissue on MMG shows as transparency. This transparent background on MMG allows clear visualization of microcalcification and any additional lesions. With ABVS, it is also possible to show this fatty degeneration: the gland appears evenly as a lobular structure of reduced echogenicity with several cord-like elements of high echogenicity, representing the thinned glandular tissue and fibrosis of supporting stroma. Usually the residual glandular and fibrous tissue is preserved in the upper-outer and central areas, while the structure of internal and lower quadrants is composed mostly of fatty tissue which is of reduced echogenicity (Fig. 4.9).

The most typical ABVS features of the breast structure at the age of 60–70 and above are an islet or narrow strips of fibrous tissue of high echogenicity and sparse ducts in the nipple and areolar areas with fatty lobules of lowered echogenicity constituting the prevalent part of the gland tissue (Fig. 4.10). So with ultrasound, we have similarity of representation compared to MMG of the fatty and fibrous tissues. As ABVS

covers the whole gland in the same projections as in MMG, it makes the ABVS images look like mammograms. Adipose tissue is hypoechoic on the sonotomogram, similar to on a mammogram. Glandular tissue and fibrosis are hyperechoic or have a denser background, as on a mammogram.

In some cases, the cellular structure of the stromal-glandular complex is preserved significantly longer, especially in lean-bodied women with a history of a long lactation period (up to 1 year) (Fig. 4.11). About 40 % of postmenopausal women have a significantly dense breast. Hyperestrogenism forms a background for the decreasing involution changes in the glands during this period. Uterine leiomyoma and endometriosis are accompanied by hyperestrogenism and hormonal imbalance, leading eventually to the stimulation of ductal and glandular epithelial cell proliferation, thus prolonging the beginning of breast involution (Fig. 4.12). Hormone replacement therapy also slows down the processes of fatty involution (Fig. 4.13).

X-ray mammography is almost incapable of detecting cancer against the background of dense glandular tissue. Meanwhile, high-density breast

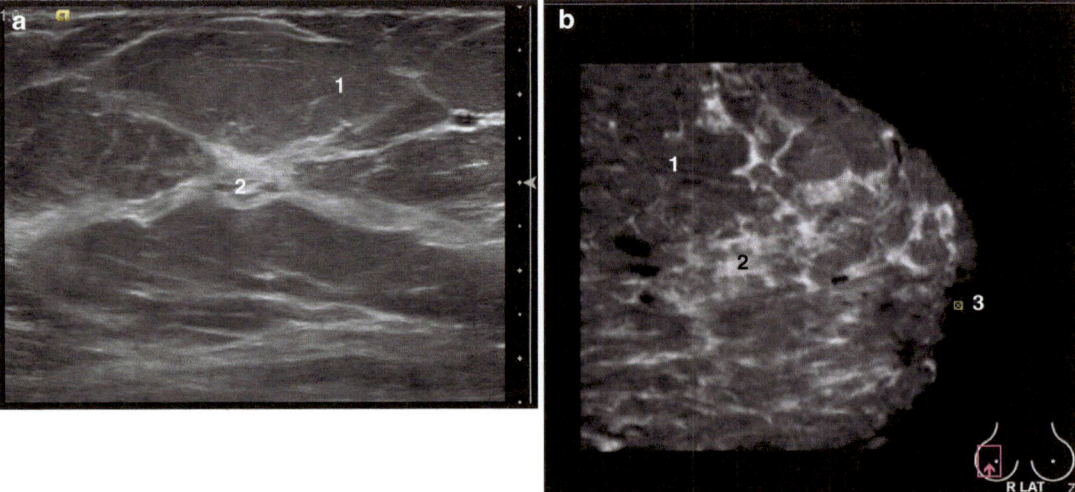

Fig. 4.9 Fat involution of the breast in a postmenopausal 56-year-old woman. Comparison of the HHUS and ABVS data for the same patient. (1) Premammary fat, (2) glandular-fibrous tissue, (3) nipple and areolar area. (**a**) HHUS image depicts the prevalence of fat tissue and thin strips of glandular tissue with fibrotic changes. (**b**) ABVS tomogram of the right breast obtained in R LAT (latero-medial view). **2** Residual glandular and fibrous tissue in the upper and central regions. In the lower ones fat tissue prevails

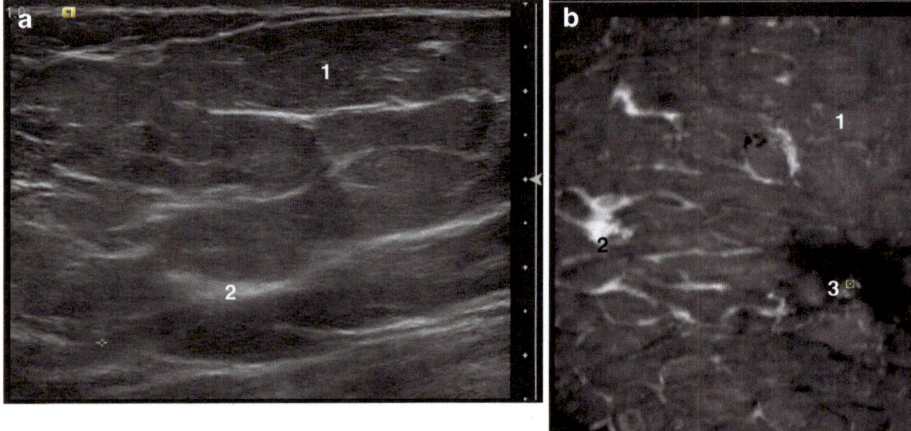

Fig. 4.10 A case study of the breast with total fatty involution in a 67-year-old woman. Atrophy of the glandular tissue. The predominant tissue is fat with a small amount of fibrous septa. Comparisons of HHUS and ABVS data for the same patient. (1) Premammary fat, (2) fibrous tissue, (3) nipple and areolar area. (**a**) HHUS of the fatty involute breast. (**b**) ABVS tomogram of the left breast obtained in AP view (coronal anteroposterior view). Uniform fatty structure of reduced echogenicity of the whole gland is seen on the coronal view

does not preclude the identification of masses by ABVS but rather enhances it [9, 10]. Therefore, ultrasound, and even better ABVS, should be present in the algorithm for screening women with dense glandular tissue (types ACR III and IV according to BI-RADS classification).

4.2   Fibroadenomas

The fibroadenoma (FA) is the most common benign breast tumor, occurring frequently in the second and third decades and being reported as a common breast lesion also in postmenopausal

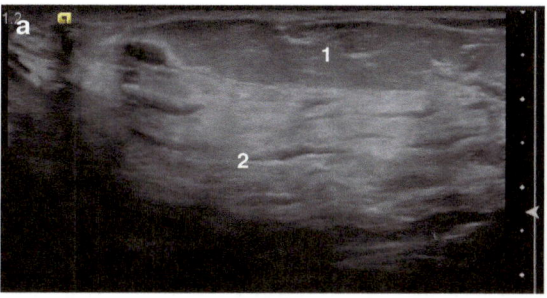
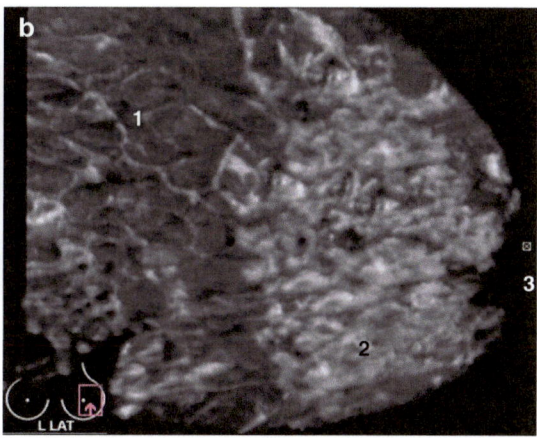

Fig. 4.11 Breast structure in a 76-year-old woman with a history of functional giant ovarian fibroma with estrogen production. The tumor caused benign transformation of the breast epithelium and slowness of the involution process. Comparison of the images obtained from HHUS and ABVS. (1) Premammary fat, (2) glandular tissue, (3) nipple and areolar area. (**a**) HHUS registered an increased amount of glandular tissue, not corresponding to the patient's age. (**b**) ABVS tomogram of the left breast. L LAT view (left latero-medial oblique view). Hypertrophied glandular and fibrous tissue in the upper and lower areas are clearly visualized

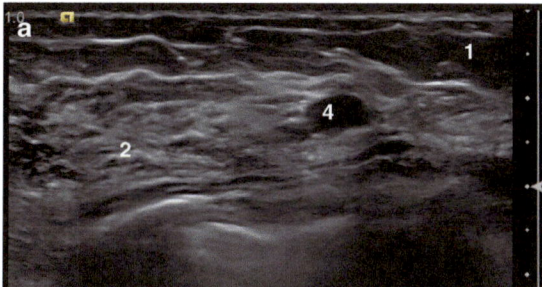
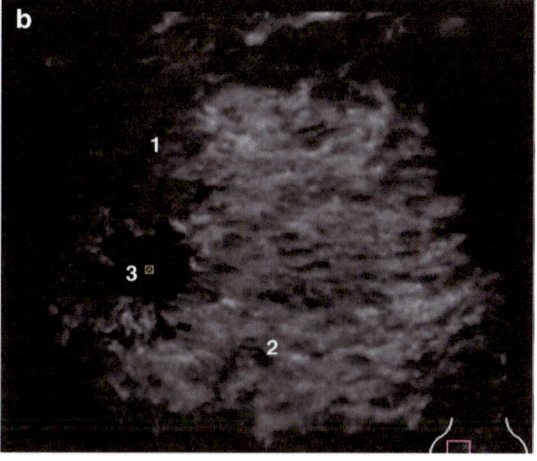

Fig. 4.12 Breast structure in a 52-year-old female who has undergone hormonal replacement therapy for 7 years. Benign fibrocystic changes in the breast. HRT slows down breast involution. Comparison of HHUS and ABVS data in the same patient. (1) Premammary fat, (2) fibrous tissue, (3) nipple and areolar area, (4) cyst. (**a**) HHUS shows thick glandular tissue with areas of benign fibrocystic changes. (**b**) ABVS tomogram of the right breast. R MED view (mediolateral oblique view). Glandular tissue with slight cellularity, no fatty involution present

women who fall into the screening age group [11, 12]. Overall fibroadenomas comprise 50% of all breast biopsies, and the rate increases to 75% for biopsies in women under the age of 20 [13]. FA often occurs as a reaction to hormonal changes. Hyperestrogenemia contributes to its development. Usually it presents as a palpable non-tender mobile lesion 1–2 cm in diameter or can be detected incidentally by MMG especially in postmenopausal women. In some patients (10–20%), they can be multiple, bilateral, or unilateral. Some FAs (especially giant FAs) can demonstrate rapid growth in adolescent girls, or during pregnancy and lactation causing asymmetry and discomfort, and thus require surgery [14]. Complex FAs are associated with an increased

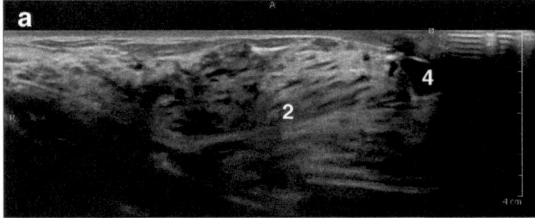 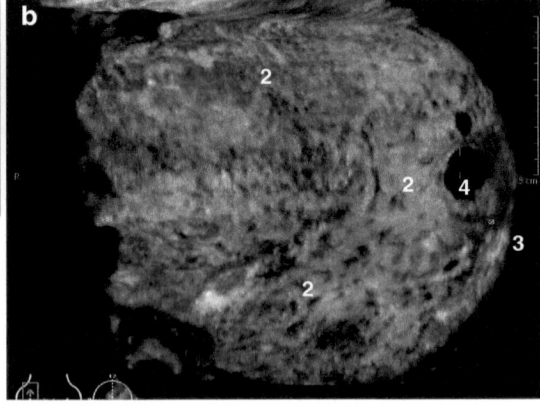

Fig. 4.13 Breast structure in a 58-year-old woman with leiomioma and diffuse endometriosis. Benign fibrocystic changes with significant glandular hyperplasia. Comparison of HHUS and ABVS. (2) Glandular-fibrous tissue, (3) nipple and areolar area, (4) cyst. (**a**) HHUS clearly depicts the increased echogenicity of the thickened glandular tissue and enlarged ducts. (**b**) ABVS tomogram of the right breast. R LAT view (latero-medial oblique view). Note an absence of pre- and retromammary fat; the reticular structure of the gland is caused by the dilated ducts. The cyst lies close to the nipple area

risk of subsequent breast cancer. Observational and molecular studies suggest FAs can transform into phyllodes tumors, which are graded as benign, borderline, and malignant.

On FNAC or needle biopsy, FAs arise from terminal duct-lobular units, the same functional unit for lobular and ductal carcinoma. An FA contains benign epithelial cells (myoepithelial and luminal). As it grows older, it becomes hyalinized, associated with calcification or undergoes myxoid degeneration. Histologically, several types of FA are defined: intracanalicular, pericanalicular, and mixed. Pericanalicular fibroadenomas are predominant in women under 45 and represent an overgrowth of connective tissue around the breast duct. Intracanalicular ones are characteristic for women over 50 and are formed inside the duct gland.

4.2.1   A Typical Fibroadenoma

Fibroadenomas are diagnosed by different methods—MMG, US, and MRI. Ultrasound is useful in diagnosis of FA. Typical US features of FAs are present in only 20–30% of cases [15]. FAs are more prevalent in young women with dense breasts in whom MMG can be negative. The US appearance of FAs includes well-circumscribed, round, or oval hypoechoic masses, slightly lobulated, with clearly defined margins, and a vessel on the periphery of the lesion or round pattern of vascularity. In hyalinized FAs, the lesion can demonstrate weak acoustic shadowing; in calcified FAs, the shadowing becomes more prominent.

Screen-detected FAs on MMG exhibit a well-circumscribed, round, or oval mass with or without lobulation, characteristically demarcated from the surrounding tissue to create a halo [16]. This is present in 98% of FAs and is caused by a radiolucent rim around the periphery of a lesion resulting from atrophy of the surrounding tissue with its replacement with fat [17]. Pericanalicular FAs demonstrate this rim on MMG more prominently than intracanalicular FAs.

The ABVS image of an FA is typical without any significant dependence on histological structure. Intracanalicular FAs are often hypoechoic and homogeneous by structure, with a clear prominent hyperechoic rim or "compression" sign. Pericanalicular FAs have a more significant echogenicity, lobulated structure, and also clear capsule or rim (Fig. 4.14). This compression sign, which is highly specific for FAs, on ABVS may be a distinctive pattern from malignant lesions which have a retraction pattern. This sign is equally well noticed in all FAs regardless of histological type in all views (Fig. 4.15).

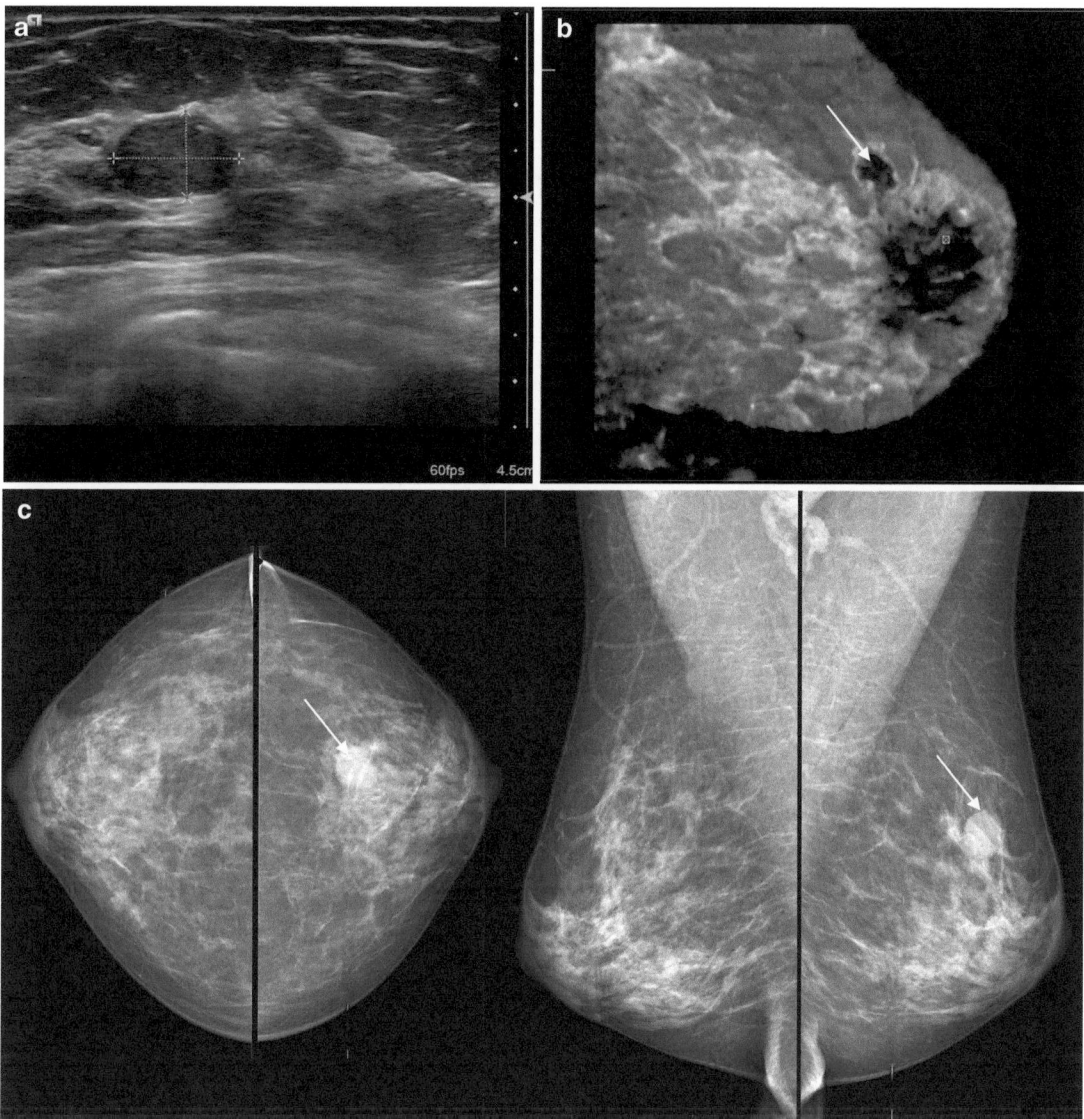

Fig. 4.14 A case of intracanalicular fibroadenoma in the left breast in a 47-year-old woman. Comparison of the data of HHUS, ABVS, and MMG. (**a**) HHUS. Fibroadenoma is presented as a clearly defined hypoechoic mass well demarcated from the echogenic glandular tissue. (**b**) ABVS. L LAT view (left latero-medial oblique view). The whole breast is seen with ABVS. A hypoechoic well-circumscribed nodule with an echogenic rim (which indicates benignity) in the upper part of the left breast can be detected (*white arrow*). The nipple is marked by a rectangle. (**c**) These mammograms (CC and MLo) of the left and right breasts are presented simultaneously for comparison. An ovoid dense mass with clear contours is visible in the upper-outer quadrant of the left breast in mediolateral oblique and craniocaudal frontal views. The lesion is marked with a *white arrow*

4.2.2   Multiple Fibroadenomas

Multiple FAs have been reported in families raising the possibility of familial predisposition. In a nonfamilial setting, multiple FAs, especially with myxoid degeneration, can enlarge in patients on follow-up leading to excision, on suspicion of malignancy [18]. The possibility of MMG to detect multiple FAs depends on their size, the presence of calcification, and the breast type (according to ACR).

Mammography shows the distinct boundary of a fibroadenoma located inside the fat tissue. It

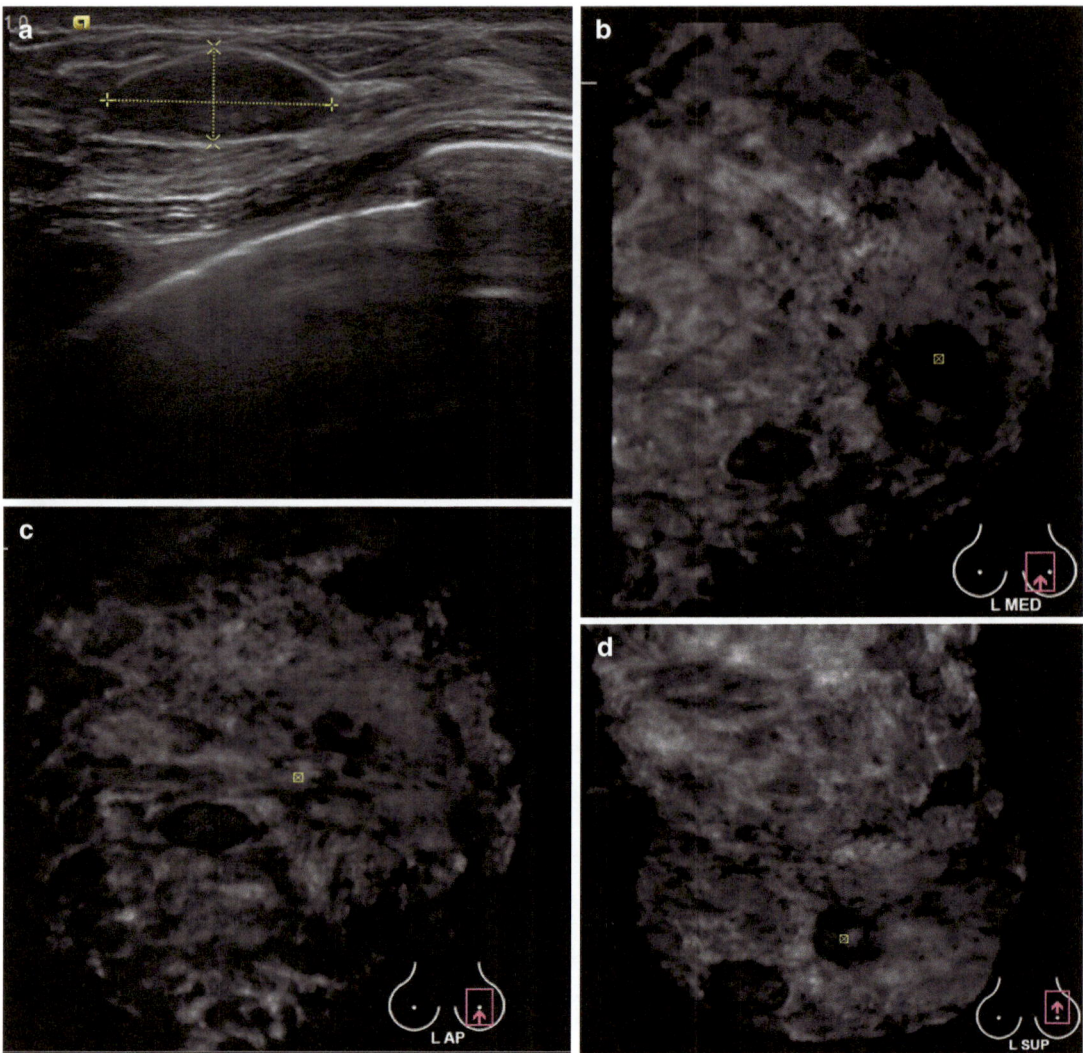

Fig. 4.15 A case of a large fibroadenoma (sized 20*9 mm) in a 35-year-old female with a dense breast. Comparison of HHUS and ABVS data. (**a**) HHUS shows a hypoechoic oval-shaped mass with clear smooth contours. (**b–d**) On ABVS obtained in different views. (**b**) L MED view (left mediolateral oblique view), (**c**) L AP view (left anteroposterior coronal view), (**d**) L SUP view (left superior-to-inferior view). "Dense breast" on ABVS is seen as echogenic cellular breast tissue corresponding to the age. Fibroadenoma in the lower-inner quadrant of the left breast, according to L SUP and L MED slices, is clearly visible on this "dense" background. A hyperechoic rim, which surrounds the FA, is thin but clear. The nipples are marked by *rectangles*

may be rather difficult to identify the same FA on a background of fibrocystic disease or dense breast. In this case, it is necessary to use the capabilities of ultrasound. US is superior to MMG due to better contrast between the FA and stromal-glandular complex. In our study, MMG failed to show a large FA in the upper quadrants inside dense breast tissue but clearly revealed only a small one—in the lower quadrants where fatty tissue dominates. Being a large one, the FA, which was approximately 2 cm in size, was occult for MMG but clearly visible for US. On side-by-side comparison of corresponding MMG and ABVS images, the large FA is masked by dense glandular tissue (Fig. 4.16). It is really difficult some times to follow up patients with multiple benign lesions. But the importance of excluding malignancy is of priority in a high-risk

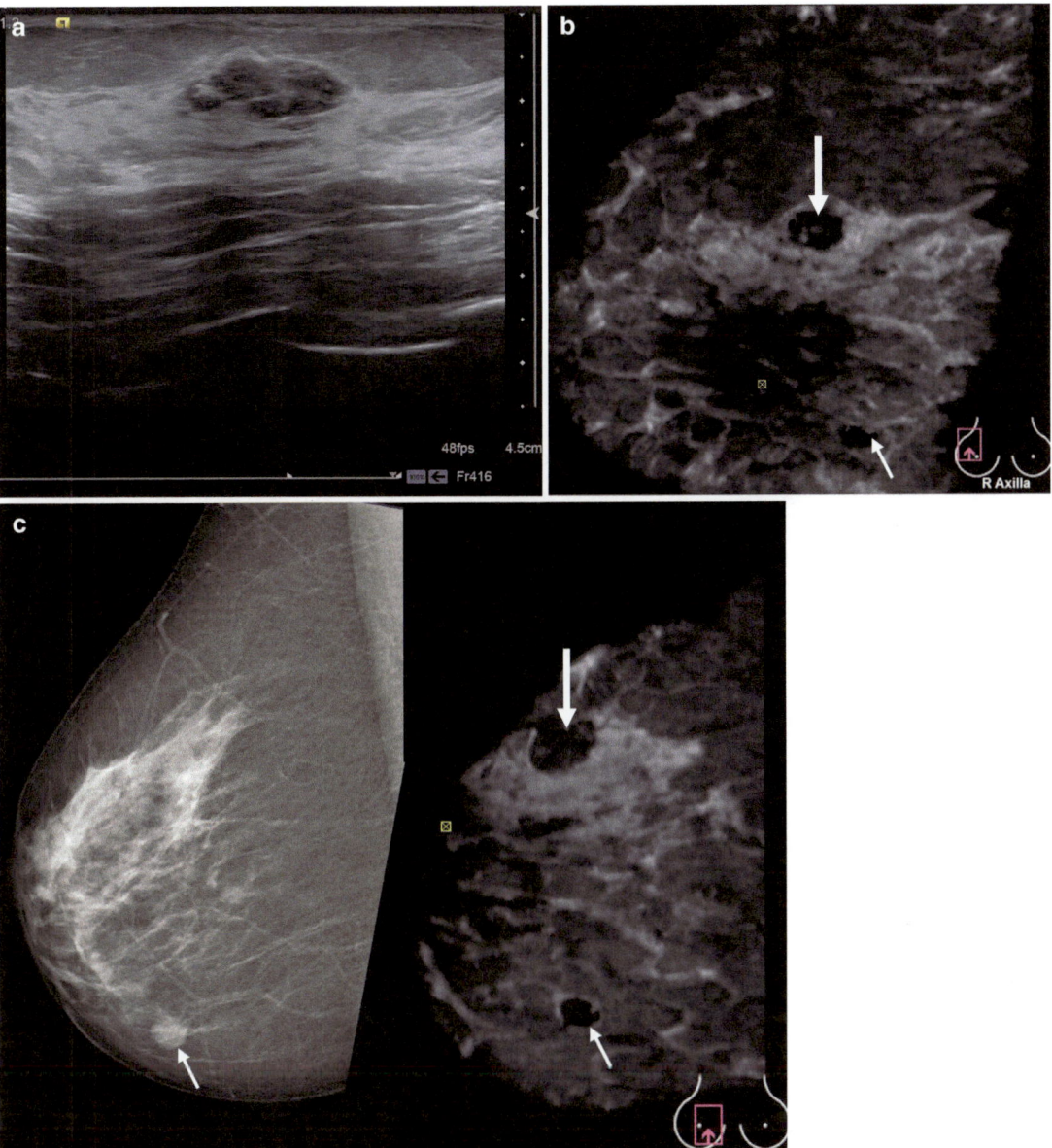

Fig. 4.16 A case of multiple fibroadenomas with an occult fibroadenoma in the upper quadrants in a 51-year-old patient. Comparison of the HHUS, ABVS, and MMG appearance. (**a**) HHUS. Hypoechoic mass with nodularity and clear margins is seen in the glandular tissue. (**b**) ABVS. RAXIL view (*axillary view*). ABVS shows two fibroadenomas in one breast in the whole gland view: one is large, and the second is small. One can be seen on the border of the upper quadrants (*thick arrow*) and the second located in the lower-inner quadrant (*thin arrow*). The nipple is marked by a *rectangle*. The residual glandular tissue is located in the upper quadrants at the 10–2 o'clock position. In other areas fatty tissue predominates. (**c**) A side-by-side comparison of the corresponding images of MMG (*left part*) and ABVS data (*right part*). MMG clearly shows only one fibroadenoma in the lower area of the breast (*thin arrow*). Dense glandular tissue with streaking and fibrosis disguises a second larger fibroadenoma. ABVS displays the fibroadenoma very clearly due to contrast with glandular tissue (*thick arrow*). Both fibroadenomas are surrounded by a hyperechoic capsule. (**d**) Image interpretation on an ABVS workstation. Multiplanar reconstruction of axillary view across a large fibroadenoma. In the left part, a coronal view of the right breast with two lesions appears; at the top of the picture, a typical longitudinal view of the lesion is presented and at the bottom a pictogram with the indication of the lesion's location at the 12 o'clock position, with an indication of the distance from the skin to the mass (1 cm) and from the lesion to the nipple (5 cm)

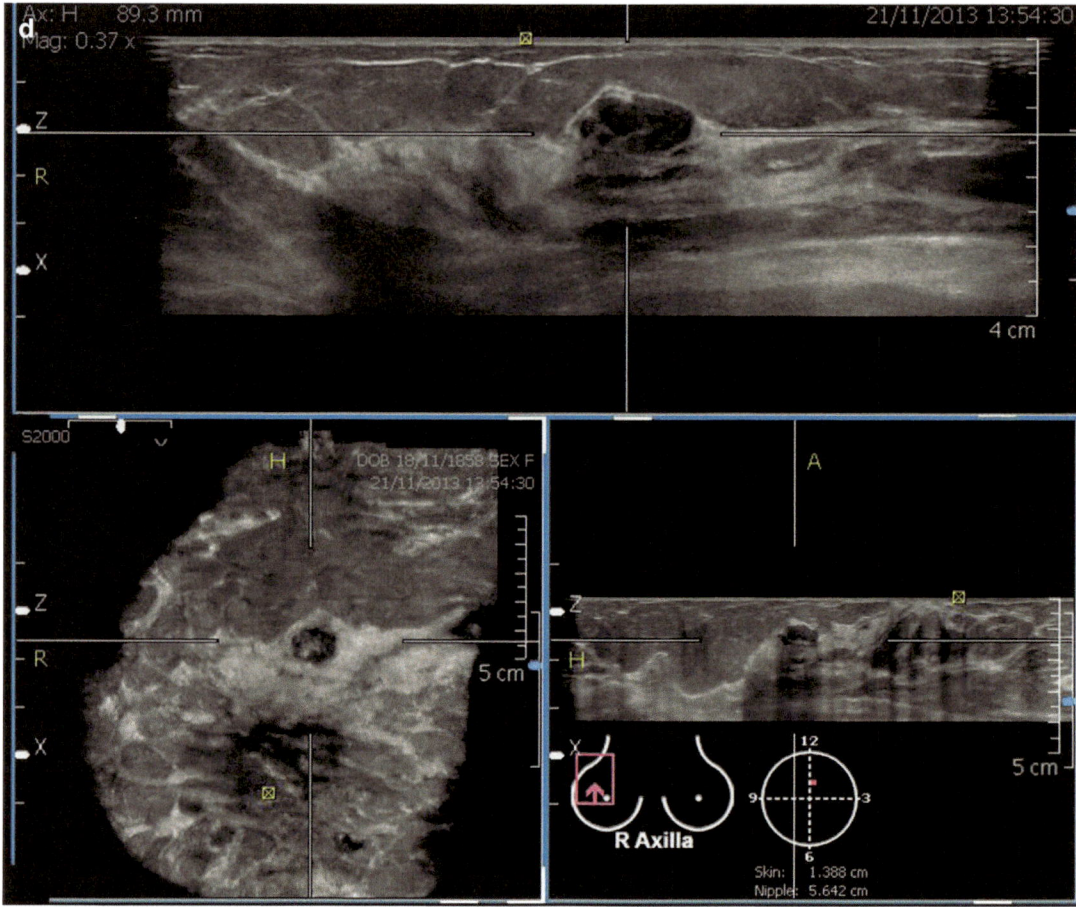

Fig. 4.16 (continued)

group of patients. In this way, the use of ABVS can help to depict all the lesions throughout the breast with better topography, size measurements, and follow-up for comparison. And in doubtful cases, the ABVS hyperechoic rim sign around multiple fibroadenomas adds diagnostic information to exclude malignancy (Fig. 4.17).

4.2.3   Calcified Fibroadenoma

Usually old FAs contain calcifications resulting from degenerative processes. An indicative sign of a long-standing FA is calcified deposits. Long-term observation may show a gradual increase in the number and size of calcifications. They are

---

Fig. 4.17 A case of multiple old fibroadenomas with a large one in the axillary recess in a 48-year-old woman simulating a multifocal cancer with metastasis in axillary lymph node on a screening mammogram. Comparison of HHUS, ABVS, and MMG performance. HHUS showed multiple hypoechoic lesions with irregular margins and a slight distal shadowing. The biggest mass (*open arrow*) was found in the axillary recess simulating an enlarged lymph node with cancerous changes. Increased superior-to-inferior diameter is noticed in the small lesion. (1) All the lesions demonstrate increased stiffness on sonoelastography, especially the large one (*open arrow*). (2) Side- by-side comparison of mammogram in MLo view (*left part*) and ABVS image (*right part*) in the corresponding R MED slice. The lesion on the MMG is dense (*white thin arrow*) with a big one thought to be a lymph node (*open arrow*) in the axillary region. In the same region, a hypoechoic lesion with a typical for fibroadenoma hyperechoic rim is noticed (thin arrow) on ABVS. (3) Side-by-side comparison of mammogram in CC view (*left part*) and ABVS image (*right part*) in the corresponding R SUP slice. The lesions on the ABVS tomogram* show a clear rim around them; no retraction sign is seen (*ABVS tomogram is not rotated clockwise)

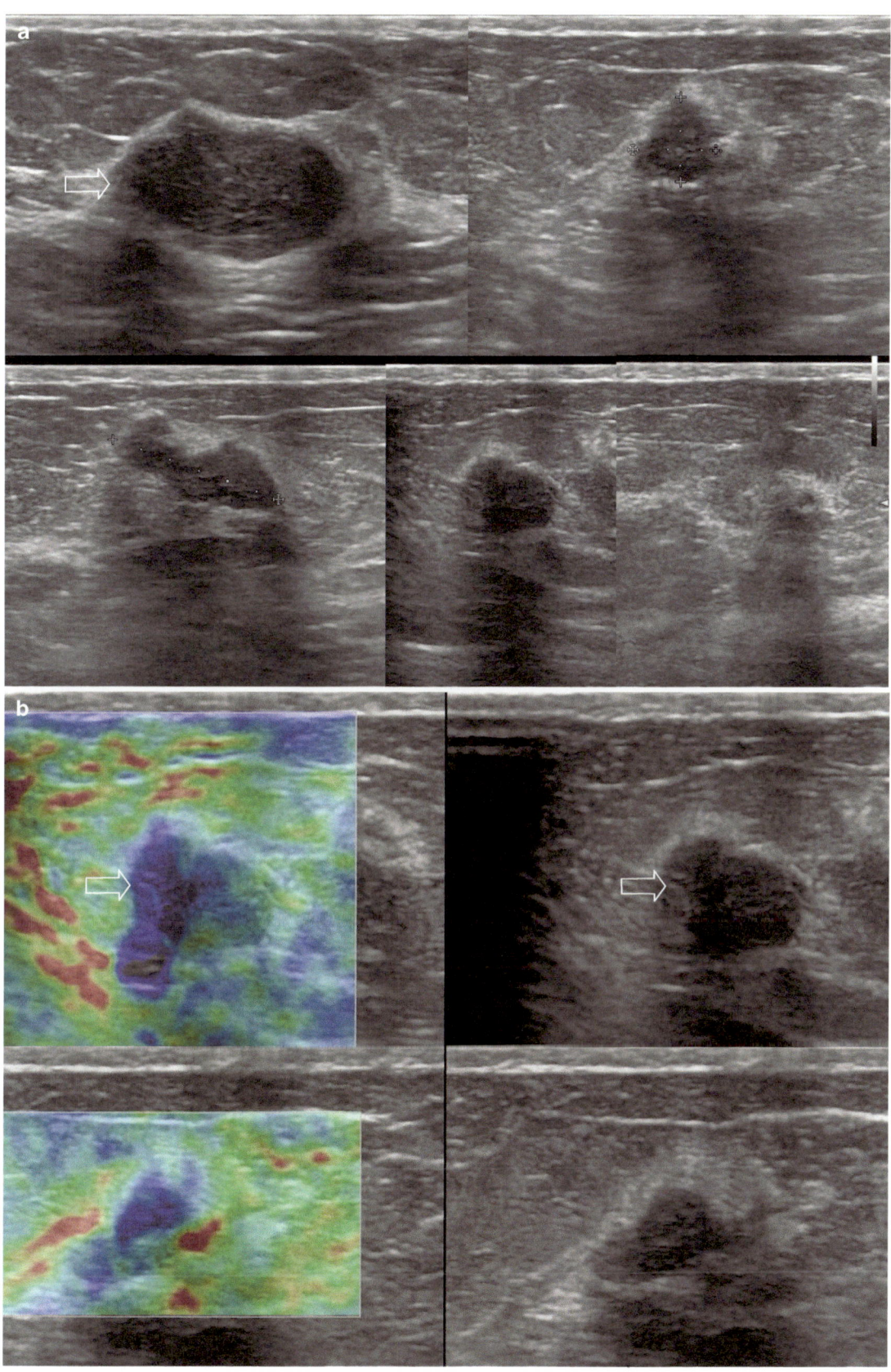

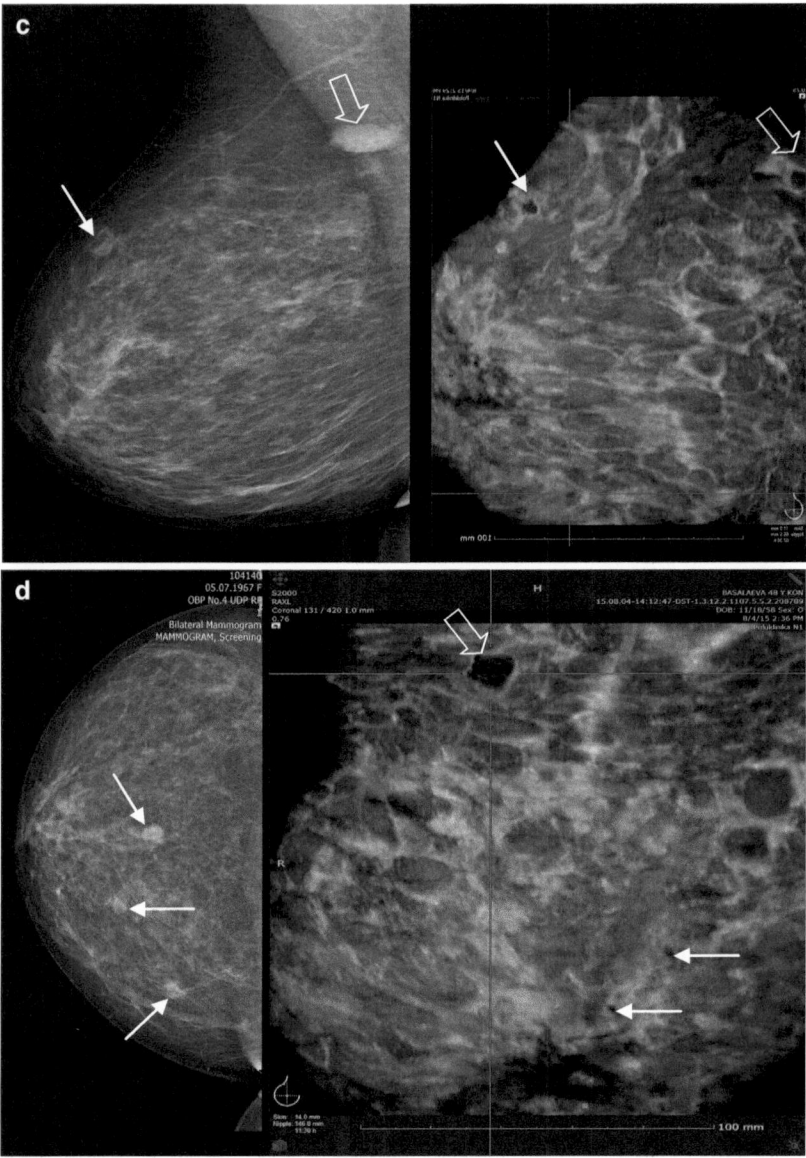

Fig. 4.17 (continued)

formed in areas of necrosis or hyalinized stroma and can be of very intricate form. A calcified FA, even a tiny one, and on a background of dense tissue, can now be easily detected by X-ray. The calcification of FA can be complete, coarse, popcorn-like bizarre calcification, evolving calcification, linear, punctate, granular, or pleomorphic [19]. The appearance of small-sized grouped calcifications on an MMG is highly suspicious in terms of malignancy and requires a biopsy, whereas a uniform benign calcification tends to require follow-up. US is inferior to MMG in depicting microcalcifications but clearly shows macrocalcifications. A distal shadowing appears behind the calcified structures. Using ABVS, it was reported that the compression sign or hyperechoic rim allows detection of the benignity of the lesions with high sensitivity and specificity [20]. The benign node on ABVS is surrounded by a thin hyperechoic capsule (Fig. 4.18).

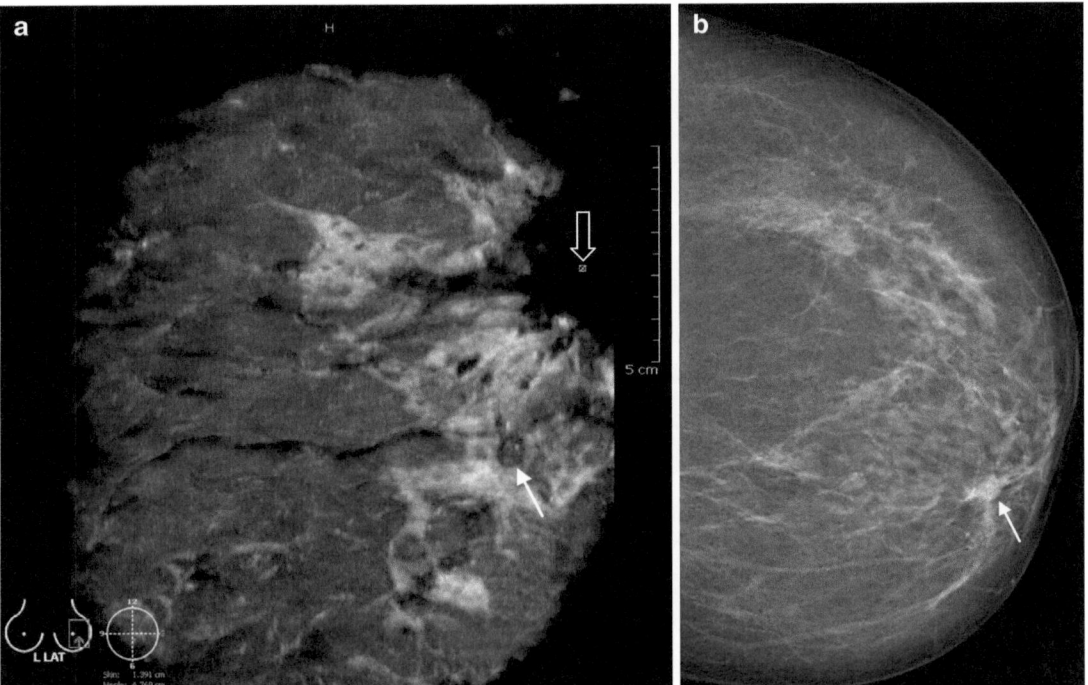

Fig. 4.18 A case of an old intracanalicular fibroadenoma of the left breast with hyalinosis of the stroma in a 55-year-old woman. Comparison of the ABVS and MMG performance. (**a**) Image analysis on the ABVS workstation. L LAT view (left latero-medial oblique view). The nipple is marked by an *open arrow*. A hypoechoic nodule with clear contours and a rim on the background of the residual glandular tissue in the central area (*thin arrow*). (**b**) Left breast mammogram in a craniocaudal direct view. Dense nodule with clear contours in the same nipple-areolar zone (*arrow*)

4.2.4 Phyllodes Tumor

Phyllodes tumor is a rare lesion which accounts 0.3–0.9 % of all breast tumors, with peaks between 45 and 49 years. It is characterized by rapid growth and large size; in some cases, it can occupy from one-half to three-fourths of the breast, varying from 2–3 to 10–20 cm in diameter [21]. The mass is non-tender, mobile, and well circumscribed. Some patients with phyllodes tumor had a past history of fibroadenoma. This tumor is characterized by a proliferation of stromal elements separated by epithelium to give rise to the frond or leaflike structures which differentiate a phyllodes tumor from a fibroadenoma. The degree of stromal hypercellularity, cytological atypia, and stromal overgrowth varies from absent in benign and low in borderline to high in malignant. The accuracy of cytological diagnosis ranges from 40 to 80 % and is not dependent on the histological structure of the tumor [22]. A low-malignancy tumor (high degree of histological differentiation) is microscopically similar to an FA and differs only by cellularity and increased mitotic activity.

Radiographically a phyllodes tumor is more typically characterized by sharp polycyclic contours and lobular structure. The signs are nonspecific. Calcifications are rare. The US picture is characterized by the appearance of fluid-filled elongated spaces or clefts inside the solid hypoechoic mass with well-defined contours. Large nodes have a lobular structure and marked hypervascularity. The ABVS picture is nonspecific and very similar to fibroadenoma (Fig. 4.19).

Suspected phyllodes tumors are better diagnosed by MRI. They are usually of homogenous high signal intensity on T2-weighted images and demonstrate rapid enhancement on dynamic contrast-enhanced MR images.

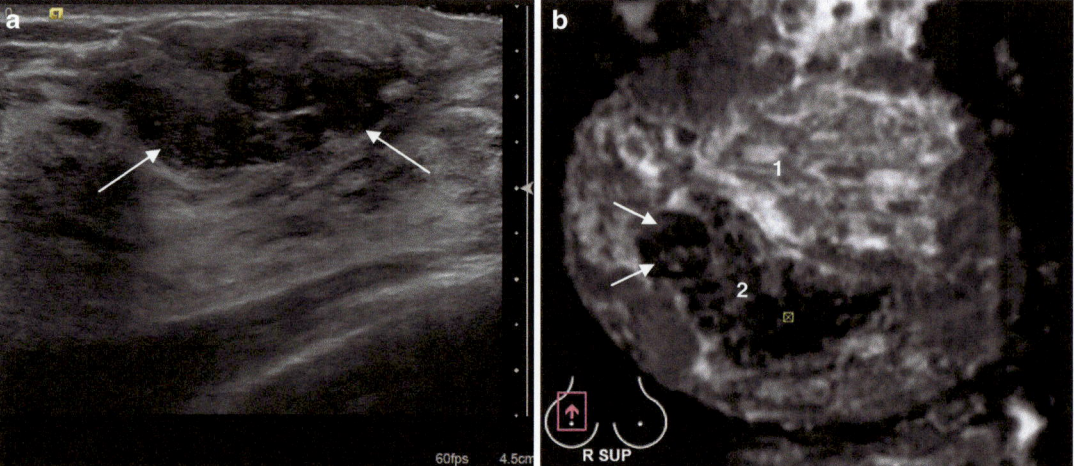

Fig. 4.19 Sonographic appearance of a benign phyllodes tumor in the right breast in a 28-year-old woman proved only after lumpectomy by histopathology. Comparison of HHUS and ABVS data. (**a**) HHUS demonstrated a large well-circumscribed hypoechoic lobulated mass with clear contours and small focus of anechoic cystic focuses inside (*arrows*) on the background of well-defined glandular tissue. FNAC found fibroepithelial cells, and histopathology has reported clefting growth pattern with variable cellularity with no mitotic activity or cytological atypia. (**b**) ABVS image obtained in R AP (anteroposterior coronal view). ABVS shows a hypoechoic mass (*arrows*) that causes the displacement of the glandular tissue (1) in the upper-external quadrant of the right breast. The signs are nonspecific

4.2.5　Atypical Fibroadenoma

A mammographic picture of a fibroadenoma often resembles those of a cyst or medullary cancer. The differential diagnosis in these cases is rather demanding. Speculation about cancer or malignant transformation of fibroadenoma is reasonable if you detect roughness of contour of the node in any place, as well as a breakthrough of the rim of clarification. The tumor may have lobulated structure, indistinct boundaries, and heterogeneous structure. Differentiation of this mass from a malignant one is sometimes difficult using both US and mammography. Mammography can change the visualization of the nodule due to the varying compression force during imaging or due to growth of the mass. Ultrasound and sonoelastography are not always convincing. Old fibroadenomas can be dense. But unlike a malignant lesion, they do not form spicules and retraction phenomenon on an ABVS tomogram, which simplifies the differential diagnosis in complex cases (Fig. 4.20).

4.2.6　Dynamic Monitoring for Fibroadenomas with 3D ABVS

Follow-up is indicated in fibroadenomas under conservative treatment. Some lesions can multiply and some progress in size with hormonal changes and several other conditions. Monitoring with US is preferable because of the absence of X-ray exposure. One can trace the growth of fibroadenomas examining their shape, documenting the exact localization of the masses, and measuring them. Reproducibility of a new method is an important factor in follow-up studies. However, HHUS is an operator-dependent technique with no possibility for independent second reading. Follow-up with ABVS resolves the tasks of independence and reproducibility. An ABVS tomogram meets these requirements. The ABVS technique is reproducible, as confirmed by publications and our research [23, 24]. ABVS data are more reliable because the scan is carried out in automatic mode; dependence on the operator and the subjectivity of the assessment are excluded.

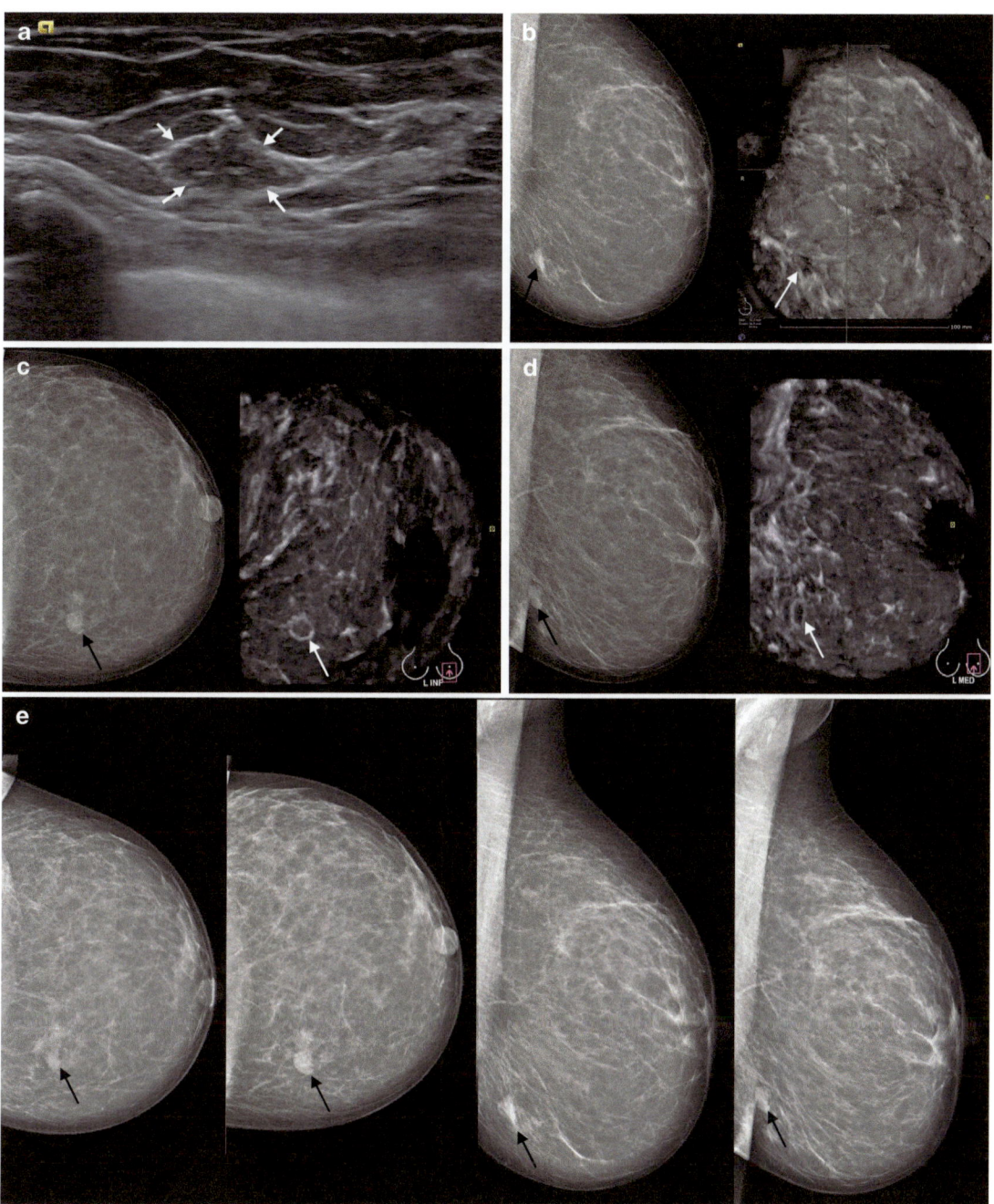

Fig. 4.20 Atypical fibroadenoma with growth changes in the lower-internal quadrant of the left breast in a 44-year-old female. Follow-up study. Comparison of HHUS, ABVS, and MMG performance. Excision with histopathology proved the diagnosis of fibroadenoma without atypia. (**a**) HHUS shows an isoechoic lesion poorly differentiated from the background of adipose tissue. (**b**) Side-by-side comparison of the corresponding images of MMG (*left part*) in MLo view and ABVS image (*right part*) in L MED view (left mediolateral oblique). The mass is considered with both techniques as an area of fibrosis. No retraction phenomenon is noticed in the area of the lesion. (**c, d**) Control study 3 months later. Side-by-side comparison of the corresponding images of MMG (*left part*) in CC view (**c**), MLo view (**d**) and ABVS image (*right part*) in L SUP (**c**) view, L MED view (**d**). The lesion has changed on MMG (*black arrow*). On ABVS it resembles a fibroadenoma with hyperechoic capsule (*white arrow*). (**e**) Series of comparative X-ray mammograms of the left breast with a 3-month interval. The changes in the dense pattern and contours are visible during follow-up

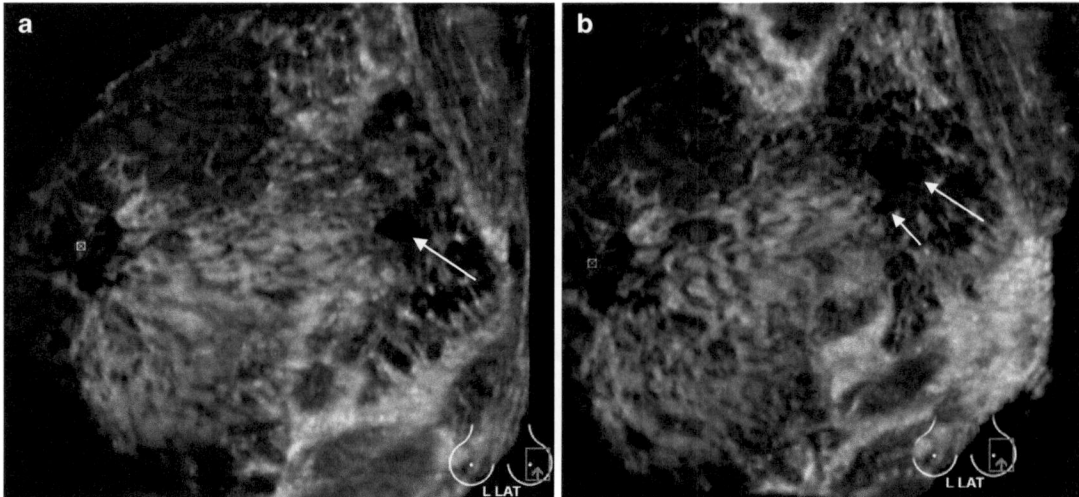

Fig. 4.21 Follow-up study of a fibroadenoma with ABVS in 27-year-old female with a history of a pregnancy and lactation 2 years ago. Comparative ABVS study of the same patient 1 year later. ABVS L LAT scans of the left breast. (**a**) Initially a single fibroadenoma is presented as a hypoechoic mass in the axillary process of the breast (*arrow*) on the background of well-defined glandular tissue. (**b**) One year later a second fibroadenoma appears in the left breast (*short arrow*). The first one is seen in the same quadrant and in the same o'clock topography

In the presented case, the patient had a fibroadenoma in the axillary process of the breast with no growth during the follow-up, but an additional small-sized fibroadenoma appeared 12 months later in the same breast, which was documented using ABVS. The absence of a small fibroadenoma in the previous study was confirmed objectively by retrospective analysis of the 3D data array from comparable views (Fig. 4.21).

Fibroadenomas more often require determination of topography of the mass to conduct a needle biopsy, so the use of ABVS in these cases is also preferred.

4.3   Breast Cystic Disease

Benign fibrocystic change is a rare condition before the age of 20 and becomes more prevalent in perimenopausal women, and microscopic lesions persist in postmenopausal women [25]. Cystic formation is most common in patients with benign epithelial proliferations and also may present in "normal" breast tissue. Benign epithelial proliferations associated with fibrocystic change include intraductal papillomas, fibroadenomas, duct ectasia, radial scars, sclerosing adenosis, epithelial hyperplasia of the usual type, and many more. Large cysts, fibroadenomas, and duct ectasia are classified as local forms of benign fibrocystic change. Diffuse forms can be represented by predominant hyperplasia of glandular tissue (sclerosing adenosis or fibrosclerosis). Diffuse and local changes can combine.

Several hormonal abnormalities have been implicated in the pathogenesis of fibrocystic change, including hyperprolactinemia, increased estrogen levels, reduced progesterone levels, and excess thyroid hormone activity [26]. The most pronounced forms of epithelial hyperplasia and cystic formation occur in patients with endometriosis. Hyperandrogenism is accompanied with a predominance of stromal fibrosis.

Apocrine epithelium is an inherent feature of fibrocystic change, and the presence of apocrine cells in a breast biopsy is generally considered by pathologists to be a reassuring feature of benignity. Apocrine metaplastic change develops in the terminal duct-lobular unit. Acini dilate because of fluid production by this apocrine metaplastic epithelium. Several adjacent acini have fused to form a larger cystic space or multi-chambered ones [27]. There is molecular evidence that some benign forms of apocrine epithelium may be potentially neoplastic [28].

Fibrocystic change and simple cysts are generally not difficult to diagnose. Usually they present in association with other screen-detected lesions.

4.3.1 Atypical Breast Cysts

Cysts can appear as round, oval, or well-circumscribed masses. Their contours are smooth and sharp. A radiolucent rim can be seen around the cyst, particularly a large one, narrow and smooth in contrast to that in cancer. Dense breasts can mimic cysts mammographically. And in fatty breasts, the cysts can exhibit the halo mark [29]. Small cysts are usually indistinguishable mammographically. The exception is the presence of calcium deposits within the cysts. Calcification is not a common feature.

Ultrasonography is the most accurate diagnostic modality in assessing cysts. Both small and large cysts are clearly visible using US. All of them have a typical appearance. Most often they are ovoid or round shaped with an anechoic content, with clearly differentiated internal and external contours, and distal enhancement [30, 31]. Sometimes cysts may require aspiration or biopsy to clarify their nature. In these cases, topographic mapping is needed. After aspiration of a cyst, follow-up US with or without MMG should be performed within a period of 4–6 weeks.

Cysts on ABVS coronal slices are found as anechoic round or oval clearly separated "cavities" without a hyperechoic rim if uncomplicated (Fig. 4.22). Fibrocystic changes are marked by the wall thickening, lumen enhancement, and roughness of contours of the ducts. "Pocket"-shaped ectasias are often detected as hypoechoic areas along the course of the main duct. These duct dilations are difficult to differentiate from cysts. ABVS can also display small cystic areas. They have a honeycomb appearance (Fig. 4.23). Dyshormonal hyperplasia can cause an increase in echogenicity of the parenchyma due to alternating hyperechoic connective tissue elements with hypoechoic glandular structures.

4.3.2 Atypical Cysts

Complex cysts are thick walled; may have thick septa, intracystic masses, or other solid components; and can also merge into a conglomerate. Clustered multiple cysts typically result from destruction of the separating septum to form a multi-chamber cystic cavity, where a part of the lysed septum can be seen. Considering the frequent multiplicity of the cysts, the question of topography arises to provide aspiration or surgical excision; and the ABVS technique can help here. An ABVS tomogram performed in "mammographic" positioning helps to determine the cysts' topography more accurately than HHUS (Fig. 4.24).

Complex atypical cysts can present with indistinct boundaries, with a lack of enhancement behind the cyst, and with the presence of internal echoes due to sediment as a result of inflammation and increased protein content, blood clots, or tumors, and therefore the cyst becomes indistinguishable from a solid mass. ABVS shows a very characteristic pattern of cysts that can distinguish them from cancer. The presence of an area of an unrimmed stamped black "hole" without "retraction" phenomenon within the breast tissue will testify in favor of cysts (Figs. 4.25 and 4.26). However, this diagnosis without a biopsy may not be safe.

Dyshormonal hyperplasia can cause an increased echogenicity of the breast parenchyma due to fibrosis. An acoustic shadow often appears behind the regions of fibrosis, obscuring differentiation of the underlying structures. Diffuse forms of dyshormonal hyperplasia should be controlled with follow-up and treated to normalize the hormonal level. In 8.5 % of cases, an overlying infection causes perifocal inflammation [30]. The mass in such patients can possess the characteristics of a malignant tumor. Wall thickening, increased vascularization in the walls, disappearance of anechogenicity, and blurring contours can require an additional examination with follow-up and sometimes biopsy.

In the following case, a 29-year-old woman presented with symptomatic painful left breast over a week and an ultrasound exam showed a tender 10*15 mm mass with stellate appearance

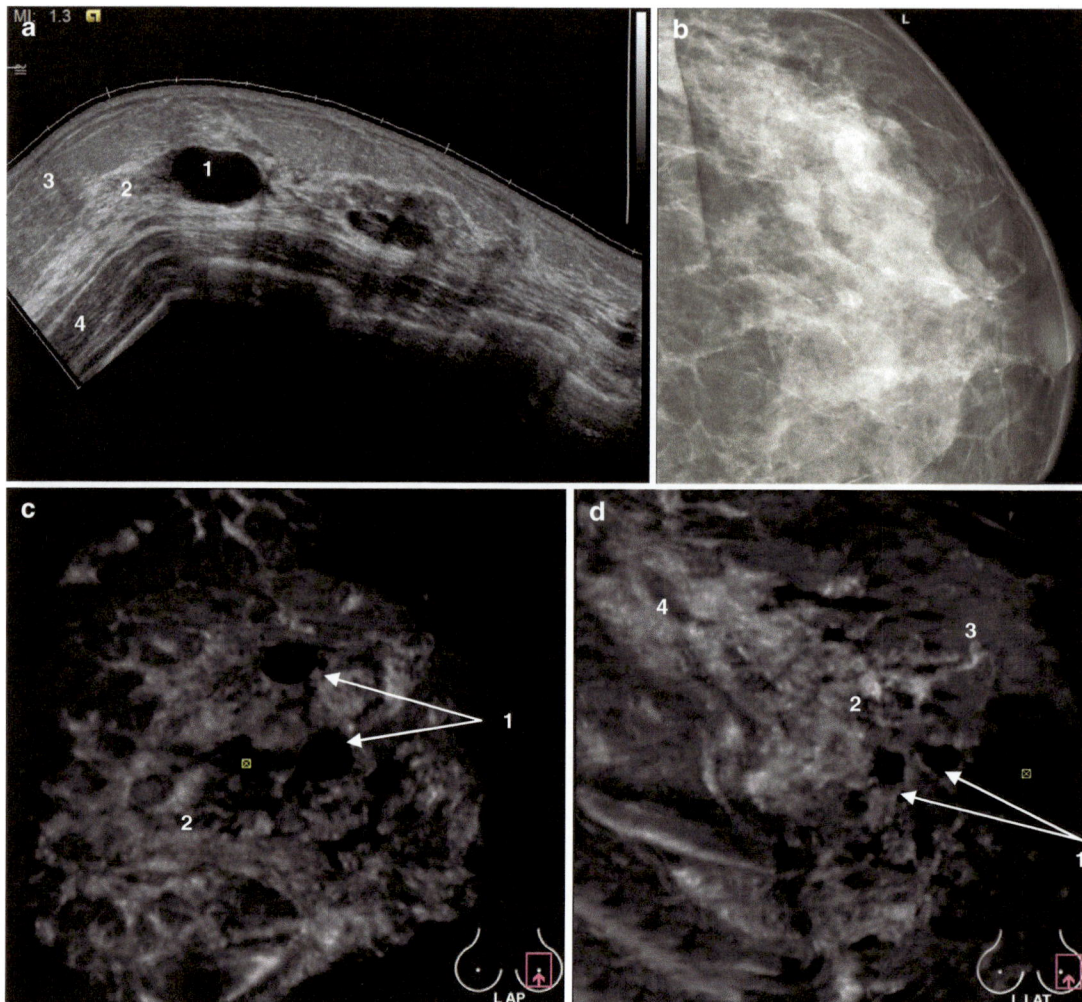

Fig. 4.22 Comparison of HHUS, MMG, and 3D ABVS data in the case of fibrocystic change of the breast in a 52-year-old female patient. Multiple cysts visualized ((1) cysts, (2) breast tissue, (3) premammary fat, (4) pectoral muscles). (**a**) HHUS. Multiple large cysts and cystic conglomerates are seen within the breast tissue. Siescape panoramic view of the breast. (**b**) MMG of the left breast. Multiple rounded opacifications in the dense breast. (**c, d**) ABVS tomogram of the left breast. (**c**) L AP slice—left anteroposterior coronal view. (**d**) L LAT view—left latero-medial oblique view. Black "holes" present in all regions on the backdrop of well-preserved glandular tissue

with thickened walls, internal echoes, peripheral vascularity, and multiple cysts throughout the breast. An ABVS tomogram showed an echo-poor mass in the upper-outer quadrant with slightly distorted contours without "retraction" phenomenon. The case was classified as BI-RADS 4 and anti-inflammatory treatment was prescribed; a follow-up exam and biopsy were recommended. The follow-up study 2 weeks later showed only multiple small cysts within the upper-outer quadrant, without areas of changed vascularization (Fig. 4.27).

A stellate pattern can appear sometimes in cysts due to fibrosis or inflammation. This can subsequently also form a spiculation on a mammogram simulating a malignant lesion. ABVS in those cases may show doubtful results which are indistinct from cancer (Figs. 4.28 and 4.29).

The frequency of neoplastic changes inside the cysts is not very high. Intracystic papillary

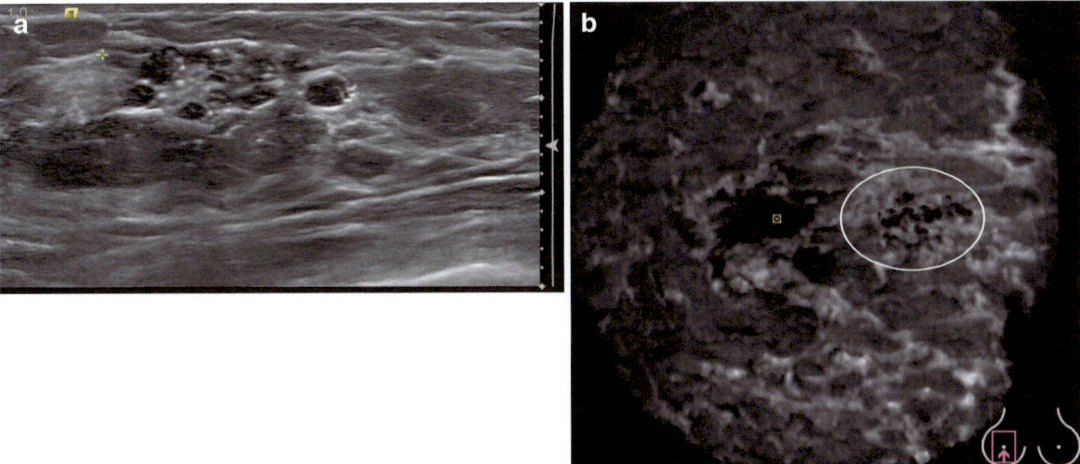

Fig. 4.23 Comparison of HHUS and ABVS performance is shown in the case of fibrocystic changes with local areas of duct ectasia in a 42-year-old woman. (**a**) HHUS demonstrates the local area of multiple cystic lesions. (**b**) ABVS tomogram of the right breast obtained in the AP view (anteroposterior coronal view) depicting the zone of duct ectasia (*circle*) in the division of inner quadrants

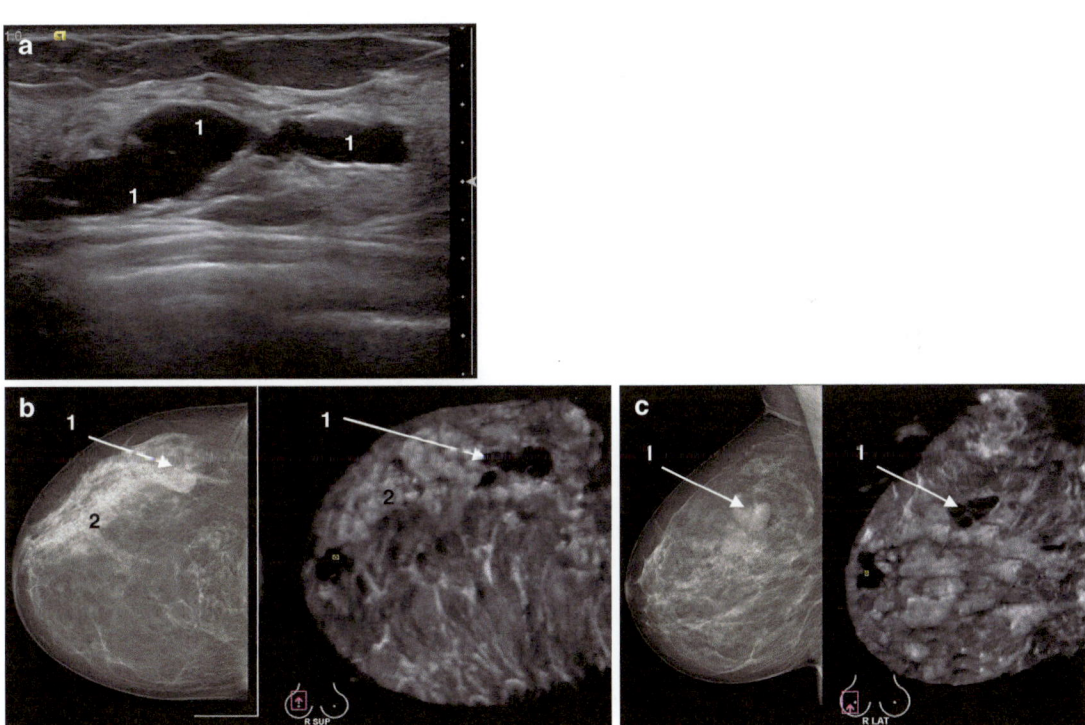

Fig. 4.24 Fibrocystic breast disease in a 51-year-old female. Comparison of HHUS, MMG, and ABVS data. (**a**) HHUS showed large cystic lesions. (**b, c**) A side-by-side comparison of the corresponding images of MMG (*left part*) and ABVS data (*right part*). Craniocaudal MMG view and R SUP (superior-to-inferior) ABVS view (**b**), MLo MMG and R LAT (latero-medial) ABVS view (**c**). MMG clearly shows the dense oval-shaped lesion on the background of dense breast tissue. ABVS differentiates this region as clustered cysts. Septations are clearly seen on R LAT ABVS image (*arrow*). Localization and the shape of the cysts are the same on MMG and on ABVS in comparable projections. Clustered cysts and dilated ducts (1), preserved glandular tissue (2) in the upper-outer quadrant

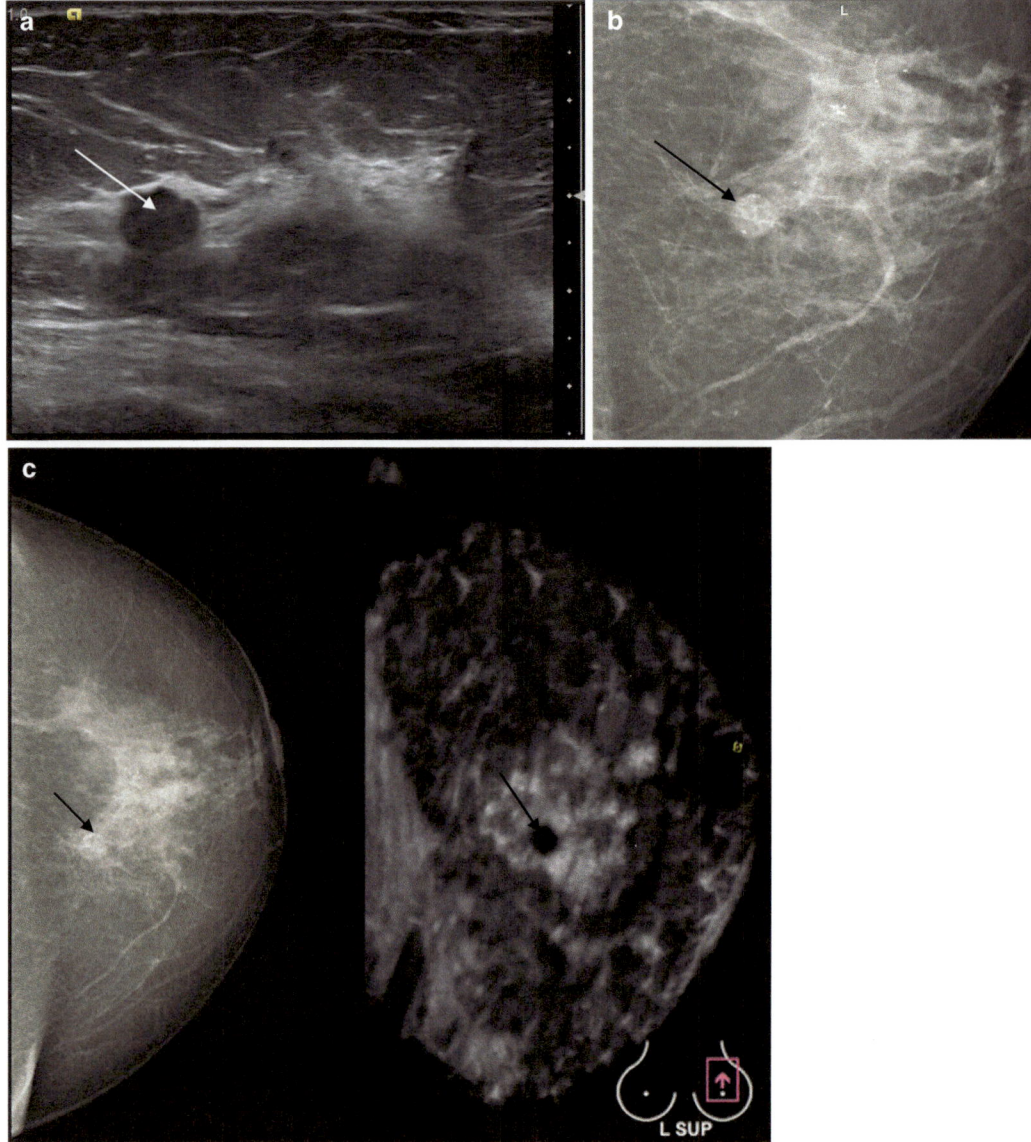

Fig. 4.25 A cyst with hemorrhagic content in a 55year-old patient with a fibrocystic change. Comparison of HHUS, MMG, and ABVS data. (**a**) HHUS. A hypoechoic mass with irregular margins and slight distal shadowing is noted. (**b**) MMG of the inner quadrant of the left breast. Dense round-shaped cystic type mass (*arrow*). (**c**) A side-by-side comparison of the corresponding images of MMG (*left part*) and ABVS data (*right part*). Craniocaudal MMG view and L SUP (superior-to-inferior) ABVS view. A "hole-like" area with stamped contours is found in the middle of the echoic glandular tissue on the ABVS tomogram, not distorting the parenchymal pattern, without a capsule and "retraction" pattern, which is typical for cysts

breast cancer is a rare pathology. Its frequency ranges from 0.28 to 0.5 % of breast cancer in general and 0.05 % of all cysts [25]. Pneumocystography was replaced by ultrasonography in assessing intracystic papillary masses [32]. Ultrasound accurately visualizes the internal papillary components and differentiates them from debris demonstrating vascularity. Malignant masses have wide basement and indistinct external boundaries. ABVS can also confirm the papillary components inside large cysts if anechoic fluid is present (Fig. 4.30).

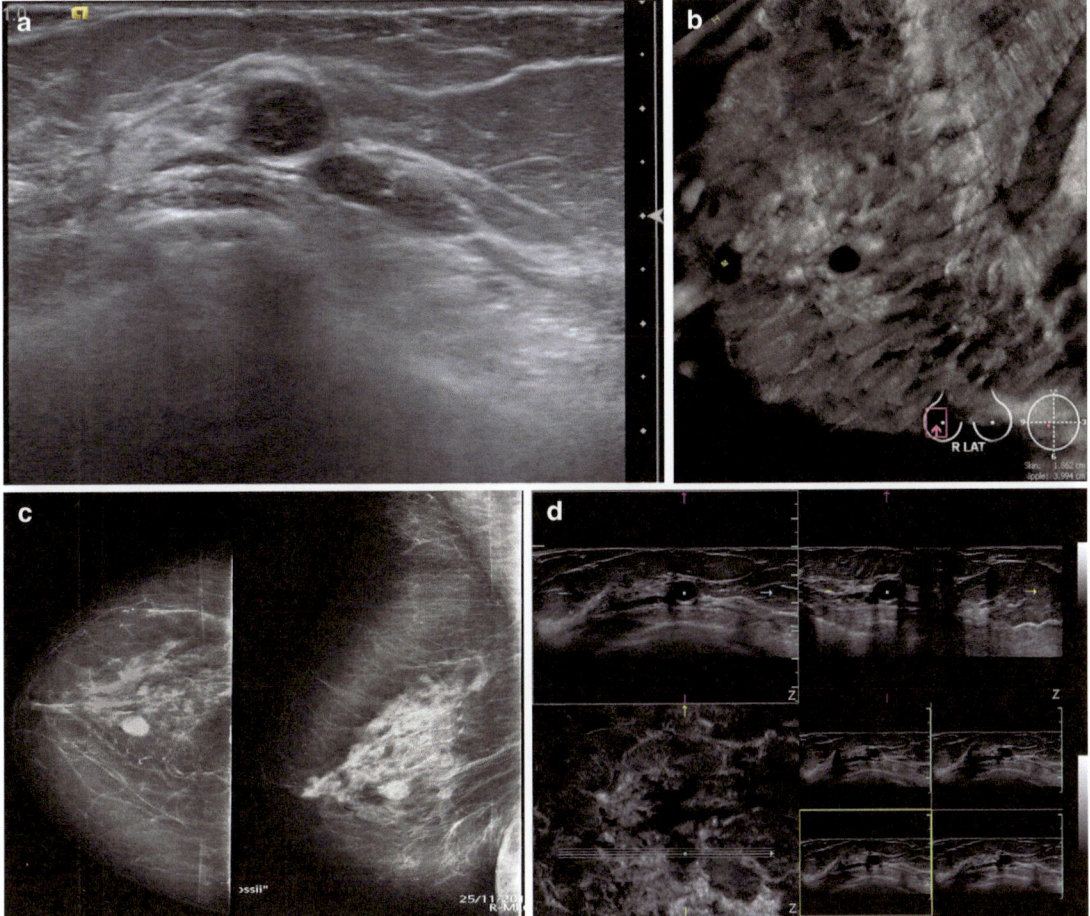

Fig. 4.26 Atypical hemorrhagic cyst in the right breast in a 59-year-old woman with fibrocystic change. Comparison of HHUS, MMG, and ABVS data. (**a**) HHUS showed a cystic mass with echogenic content. (**b**) ABVS image analysis on the workstation of the R LAT slices (right latero-medial view). Anechoic structure with smooth con- tours without distinct rim. (**c**) Mammograms of the right breast CC and MLo views. Dense round mass in the cen- tral part of the right breast. (**d**) ABVS image in multipla- nar reconstruction mode performed on the US device. Cross-sectional view through the cyst

Multiplanar reconstruction or slice-by-slice previewing through the cyst easily reveals cysts with solid lesions.

4.4   Breast Cancer

Breast cancer is common in women and a leading cause of cancer mortality in women worldwide [33]. Early preclinical diagnosis is of significant value because the sooner a tumor is detected, the longer the life expectancy of the patient. Life expectancy in breast cancer is influenced by the tumor size, presence or absence of metastases in regional lymph nodes, presence of receptors to female sex hormones in the tumor, histological type of the tumor, and many other factors. The number of such factors is growing as tumor biol- ogy is studied. Breast cancer is a heterogeneous disease with variations in morphological picture, clinical course, and sensitivity to treatment. This is due to the differences in tumor biology at the molecular level. The most aggressive are TN (triple-negative) and HER2-positive carcinomas. The most common histological type is consid- ered to be ductal carcinoma, less common are

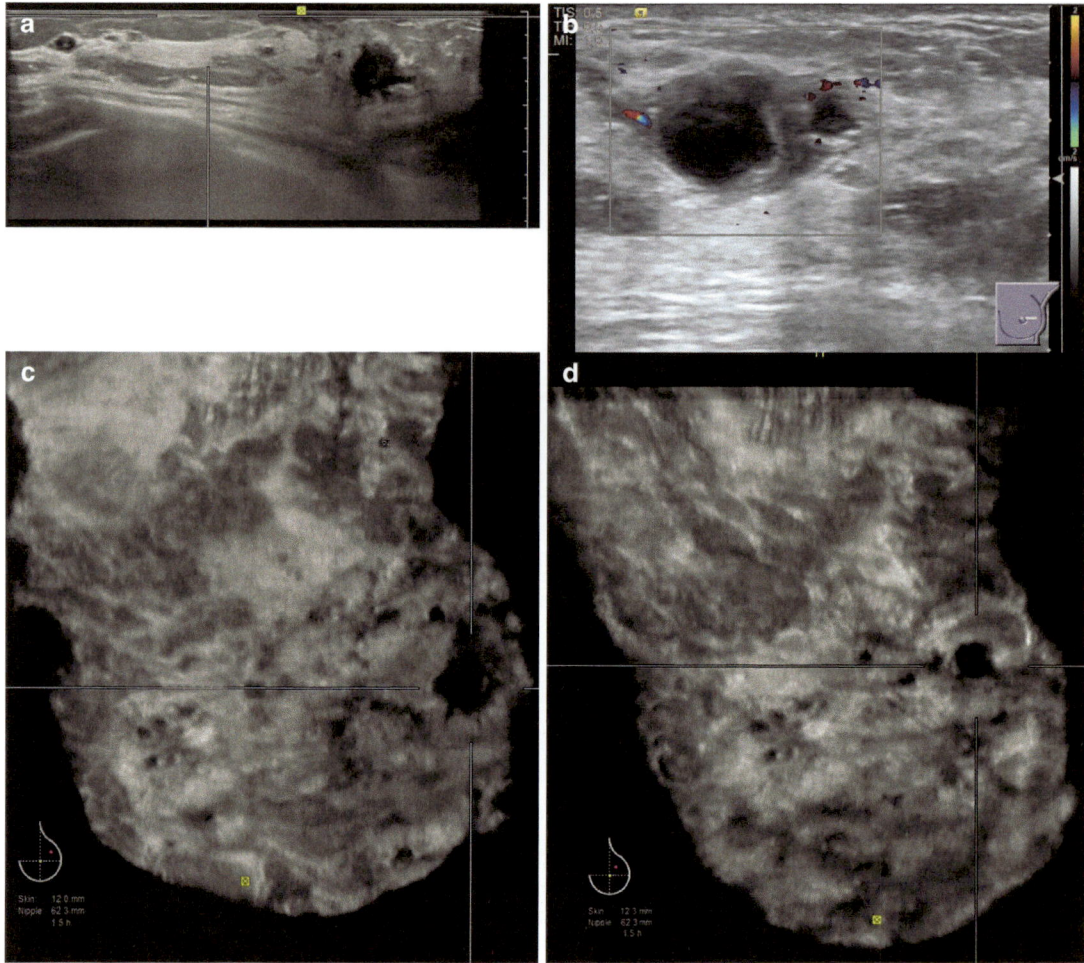

Fig. 4.27 Follow-up study of non-lactation mastitis with a complex cyst in a 29-year-old patient. The aspirate consisted of thick material resembling pus. The cytology showed numerous macrophages in an amorphous background. No epithelial cells or malignant cells are seen. Comparative results of HHUS and ABVS data ((**a–c**) US study before treatment, (**d**) follow-up study after the treatment). Explanation in the text. (**a**) Gray scale HHUS. (**b**) HHUS in color Doppler mapping (CDM). (**c, d**) ABVS images of the left breast

lobular, mixed, medullary, colloid, nipple, and others. The numerous types of breast tumor cause polymorphism of their clinical, mammographic, and sonographic manifestations. The stage of the tumor is directly related to its size and spread. Therefore, any diagnostic method should not only identify the primary tumor but also assess the extent it has spread.

Therefore, the interest in developing new methods of early and specific diagnosis of nonpalpable and "minimal" breast cancers of less than 1 cm is growing. X-ray mammography is established as a "gold standard" for assessing breast structure and breast density and for identifying regional axillary lymph nodes. MMG screening reduces mortality from breast cancer by more than 30 % [34]. However, the sensitivity of mammography depends on the breast density. Studies on women with dense breasts have demonstrated a sensitivity of MMG of less than 50 % [35]. More than 50 % of women younger than 50 and at least one-third aged over 50 have been found to have dense breast tissue [36]. Thus, cancer will be missed mammographically in every second woman with a dense breast. A mammogram is a summation

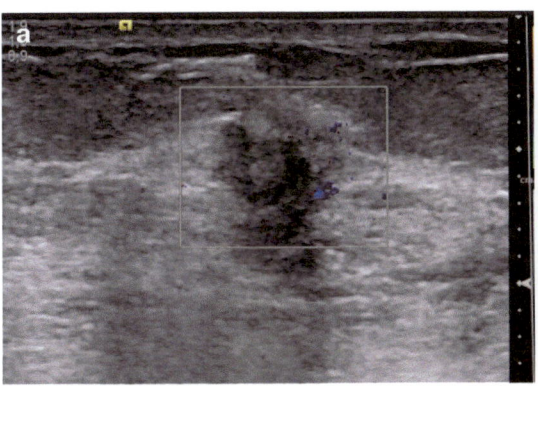

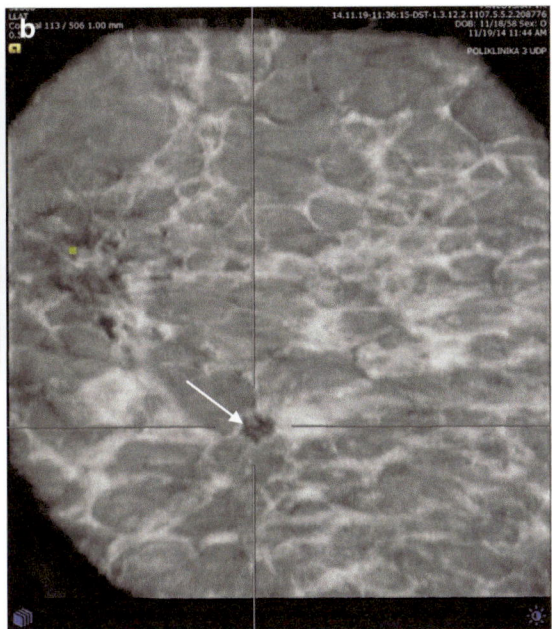

Fig. 4.28 A case of a complex cyst with contents which simulate a malignant lesion. Comparison of HHUS and ABVS data. (**a**) HHUS in Color Doppler mode. A mass with irregular contours, sized up to 10 mm, with visible distal acoustic shadowing and perinodular vasculariza-tion. (**b**) ABVS image obtained in LAT view (latero-medial oblique). An undulating contour simulates "retraction" phenomenon (*arrow*). The biopsy showed a bloodstained substance with apocrine metaplasia, without atypia

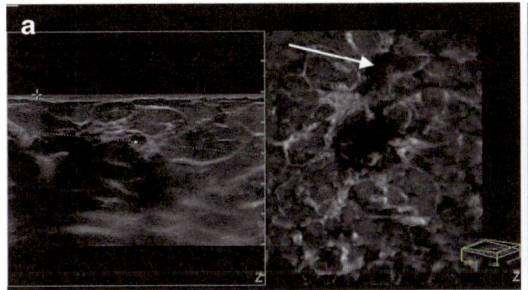

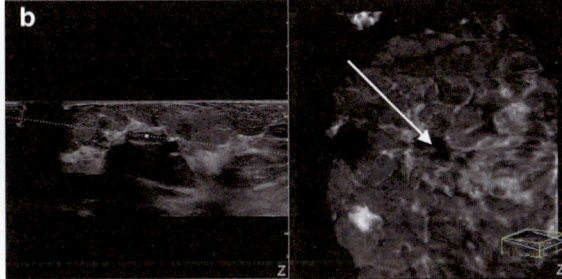

Fig. 4.29 A case of a cyst with previous inflammation in a patient with a fibrocystic change. Histopathology revealed stromal hyalinosis and leukocyte infiltration; no atypical cells were found. (**a**) ABVS obtained in AP view (anteroposterior). Multislice view through the lesion based on the sagittal slice (*right part*), perpendicular coro-nal slice of the same lesion (*left part*). A spiculation pat-tern is presented on the coronal view of the lesion corresponding to the zone of postinflammatory changes and cystic rearrangement (*arrow*), simulating a malignant pattern. (**b**) ABVS. Multislice view through the lesion based on the axial slice (*right part*), perpendicular coronal slice of the same lesion (*left part*). The hypoechoic region with spiculation on the coronal slice is presented in the zone of postinflammatory changes

image with all breast tissue overlapping in each view, thus resulting in missed cancer. It was found that the odds of interval cancer among women with extremely dense breasts were 17.8 times greater than among women with fatty breasts. In addition, breast density has been established as an independent risk factor for breast cancer [9].

Breast ultrasound, as currently considered among breast imaging modalities, has an essential

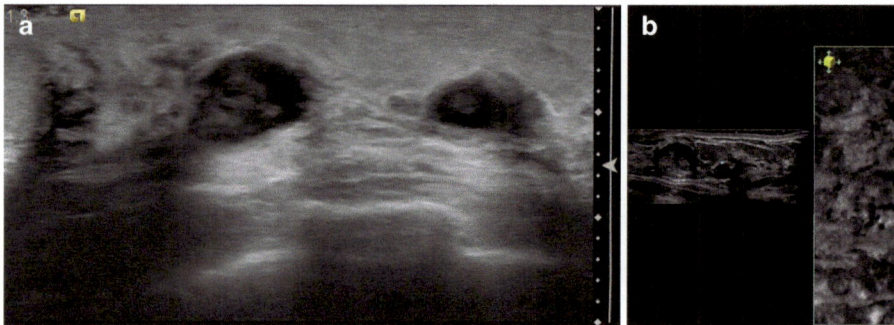
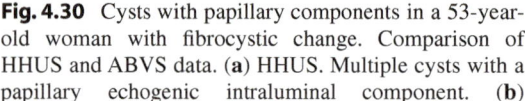
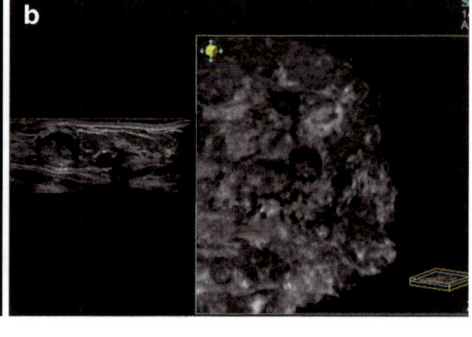

Fig. 4.30 Cysts with papillary components in a 53-year-old woman with fibrocystic change. Comparison of HHUS and ABVS data. (**a**) HHUS. Multiple cysts with a papillary echogenic intraluminal component. (**b**) ABVS. Multislice view through the lesion (*right part*), latero-medial oblique slice perpendicular to the sagittal slice (*left part*). Papillary components are visible inside the cysts not altering the outer contours of the cysts

and specific role as a complementary method to mammography for woman with dense breasts and clinically or radiologically detected suspicious breast lesions [37]. A combination of mammography with ultrasound in women after 40 with radiographically dense breasts doubles the detection of cancers [38, 39]. HHUS represents the gold standard for examination of young patients in which mammography is not indicated because of exposure of the breast to ionizing radiation and risk of induced breast cancer. However, the dependence on the operator for HHUS is a major concern with respect to the widespread use of whole-breast US.

Automated breast volume imaging has several advantages over HHUS: the technique is more reproducible, has 3D capability with multiplanar reconstruction, and allows delayed interpretation outside real time, optimizing the radiologist's reading environment [40]. ABVS provides additional information to radiologists about breast cancer, especially in women with dense breast. A coronal view of the entire volume offers an easily understandable representation of the global breast anatomy and architecture, and also helps surgeons, giving a comprehensive sight of the breast from the skin line to the chest wall [23]. Breast cancer, especially IDC, shows a "retraction" phenomenon on ABVS coronal views, which is valuable in differentiating lesions as malignant [41, 42]. The high sensitivity of ABVS in detection of breast cancer was shown in many studies [23, 43–47].

4.4.1 Spiculated Breast Cancers

Cancer has a very typical stellate pattern on a mammogram, with a central dense region with uncircumscribed margins, which extend into the surrounding tissue as several gradually tapering strands. They are formed as a result of desmoplastic reaction around the tumor and periductal fibrosis. The spiculation of the tumor, "retraction" phenomenon, and "radiance" are features of malignancy. These changes are usually visible on X-ray MMG. But sometimes overlapping effect and increased breast density masks this sign. In these cases, additional methods of examination are needed, for example, X-ray digital breast tomosynthesis, which helps to identify a tumor site more accurately by obtaining a series of subsequent breast images. The alternative is ultrasound examination. However, before the era of 3D breast ultrasound, it was not always possible to see this phenomenon using conventional 2D ultrasound. Various artifacts, while they mechanically collected US volumetric data, precluded the full identification and assessment of the significance of the findings in the diagnosis of breast cancer. ABVS technology is able to detect this phenomenon. The dimensions of the tumor and molecular type of the tumor do not affect the severity of the symptoms. The "retraction" symptom is clearly seen even in nodules less than 5 mm [48, 49]. Around the tumor, a hyperechoic halo develops as a crown, with a hypoechoic central zone (Fig. 4.31).

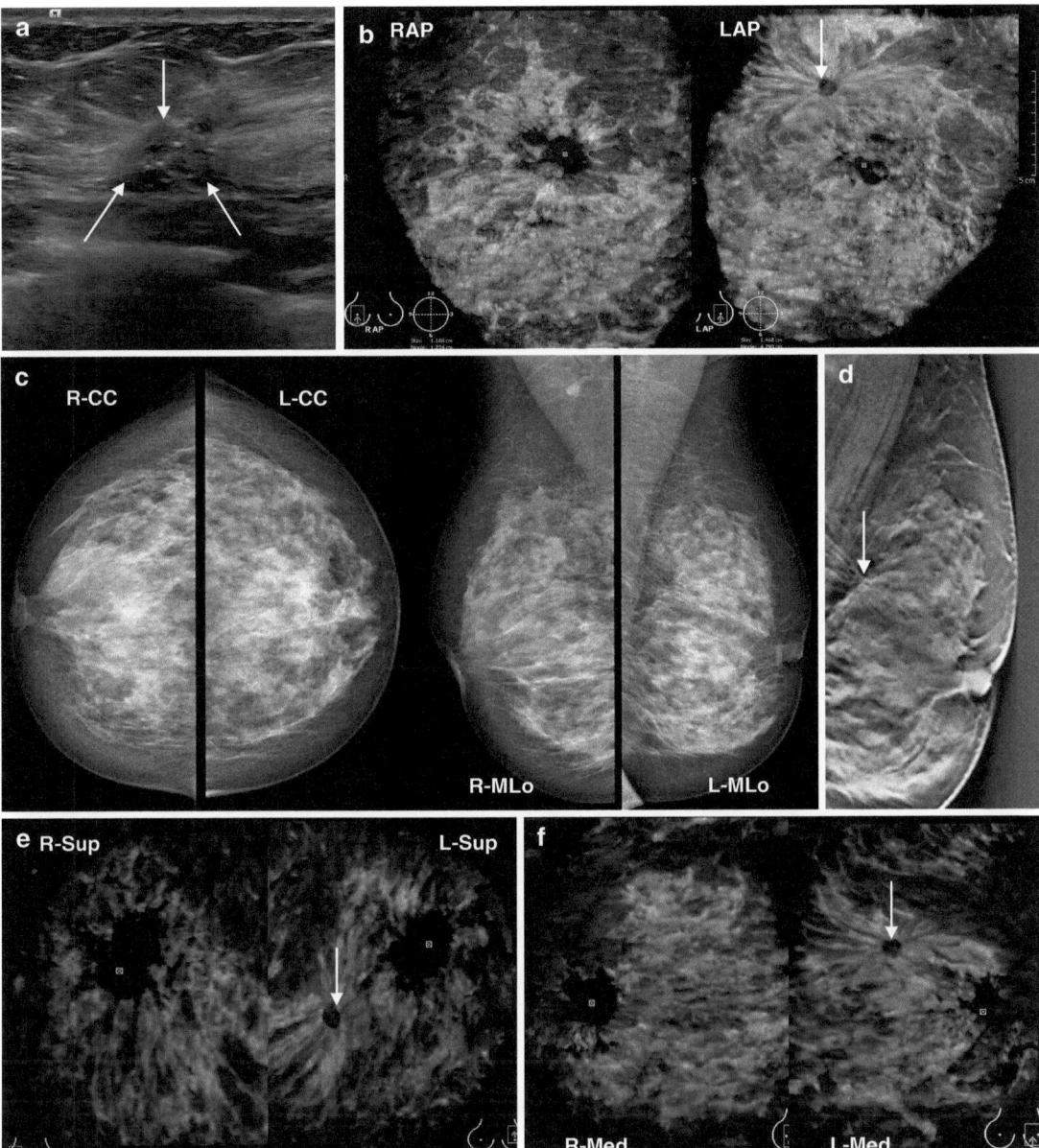

Fig. 4.31 Invasive ductal carcinoma in the upper-inner quadrant of the left breast in a 50-year-old female not found with palpation. Histopathology, immunohistochemistry: T1aN0M0, TN, grade G1. Multimodality study. Comparison of HHUS, ABVS, MMG, DBT findings. (**a**) Gray scale HHUS shows the tumor nodule less than 1 cm with irregular margins and microcalcifications lying within the hyperechoic breast fibrous tissue (*arrows*). (**b**) On bilateral ABVS of right and left breasts, an asymmetry is noted on coronal projections (R AP and L AP). In the upper-inner region of the left breast, a hypoechoic lesion with severe retraction phenomenon is seen (*arrow*). (**c**) Mediolateral oblique and craniocaudal bilateral breast mammograms (R-CC and L-CC; R-MLo and L-MLo) show a heterogeneously dense breast with no discernible abnormality. The cancer was missed by MMG due to dense breast and the particular localization of the tumor (upper-inner quadrant). (**d**) Digital breast tomosynthesis of the left breast in mediolateral oblique projection reveals the subtle tumor nodule with severe spiculation (*arrow*). (**e, f**) Bilateral ABVS. Side-by-side comparison of the symmetrical projections (**e**) R-Sup (*left part*) and L-Sup (*right part*); (**f**) R-Med (*left part*) and L-Med (*right part*). The tumor nodule with spiculation is clearly visible on both views (*arrow*)

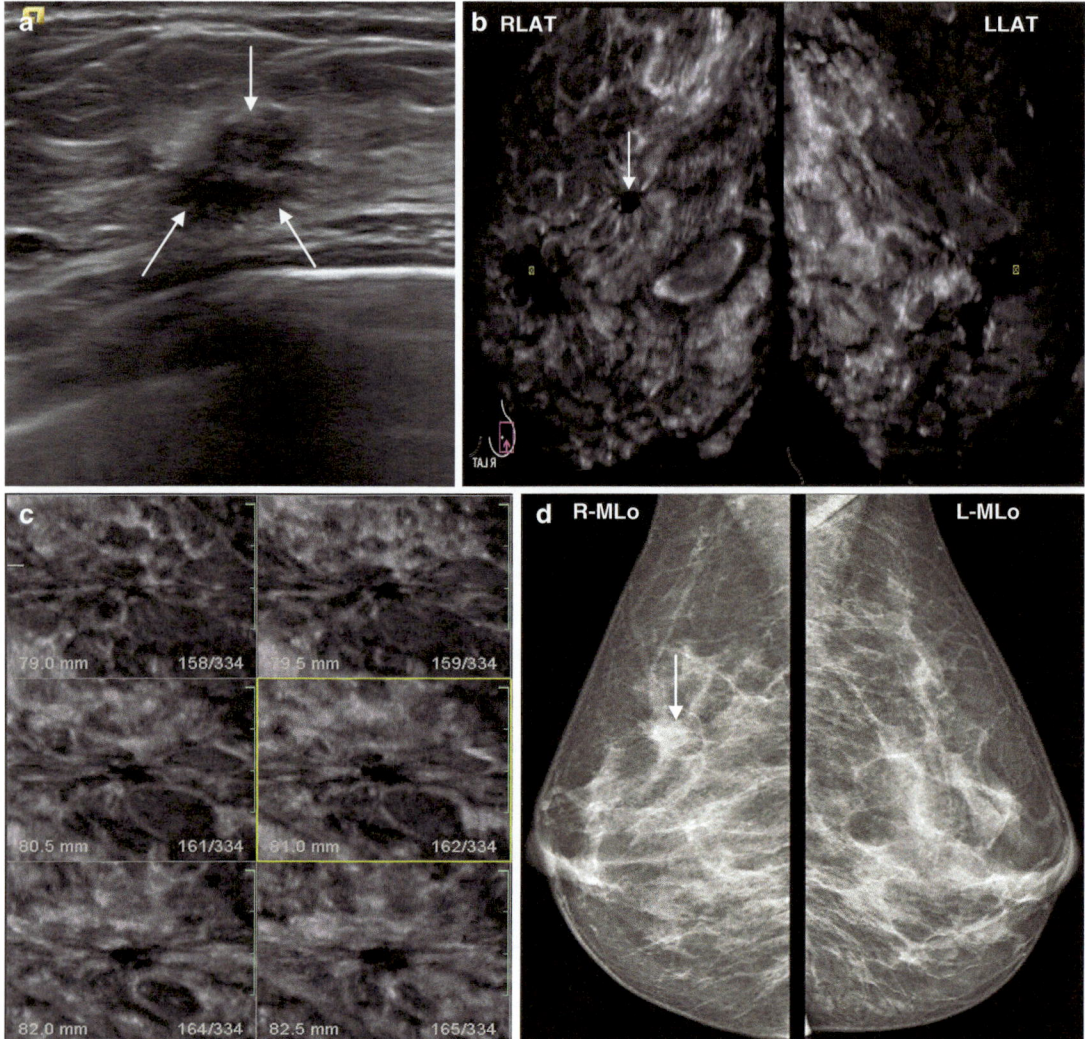

Fig. 4.32 A 44-year-old woman with palpable abnormality in the upper-outer quadrant of the right breast. Histopathology proved IDC, T1aN0M0, luminal type A, grade G2. Comparison of the performance of HHUS, ABVS, MMG. (**a**) A hypoechoic nodule less than 1 cm with echogenic halo and indistinct boundaries with increased anteroposterior size is seen on HHUS (hyperechoic halo caused by desmoplastic reaction). (**b**) Bilateral ABVS tomograms. Comparison of R-Med (right mediolateral oblique—*left part*) and L-Med (left mediolateral oblique—*right part*) projections. The lesion with spiculation effect is clearly visible in the right gland (*arrow*). (**c**) A multislice view with creation of serial sections through the tumor obtained by ABVS. Coronal slices of the tumor with a 1 mm slice thickness. The "retraction" phenomenon is clearly visible. (**d**) Bilateral MMG. Side-by-side comparison of MLo views (R-MLo and L-MLo). The nodular density in the upper part of the right breast is more prominent within the dense breast (*arrow*)

The "retraction" phenomenon is characteristic for 90 % of breast cancer cases. A. Broberg et al. (1983) noted that the nodes with spicules usually occur in women with a high content of estrogen receptors in the breast [50, 51]. However, we have not noted any clear relationship of their content with the histological grade of differentiation and molecular type of the tumor. All cases of basal and luminal type A cancer demonstrated this sign, and in luminal type B and Her2neu overexpressing tumors, this sign was observed in 80 % of cases (Fig. 4.32).

This "retraction" phenomenon allows one to differentiate between benign and malignant nodules under questionable characteristics in B-mode and advanced US angiography and

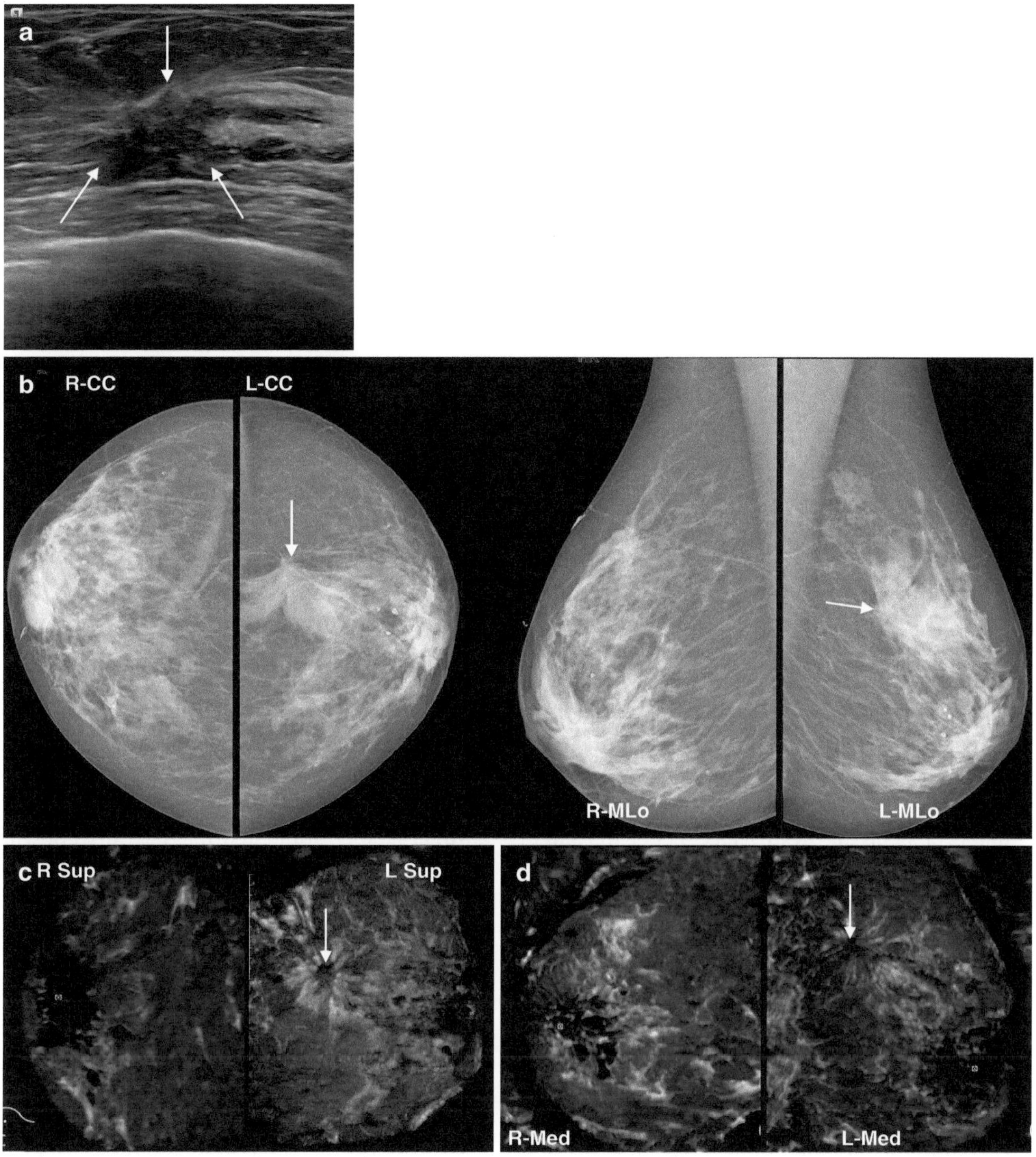

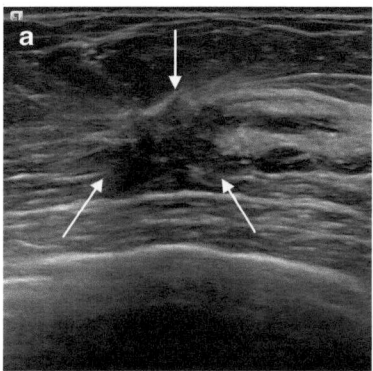

Fig. 4.33 A 44-year-old female patient with a palpable upper internal quadrant mass in the right breast. IDC, T1N0M0, luminal type B, grade G3. Comparison of the HHUS, MMG, ABVS. (**a**) Stellate hypoechoic tumor less than 1 cm within the residual glandular tissue (*white arrows*). (**b**) Side-by-side bilateral mammograms in CC and MLo projections (R-CC and L-CC; R-MLo and L-MLo). Architectural asymmetry due to significant "retraction" phenomenon in the dense breast (*black arrow*). (**c, d**) Bilateral breast ABVS tomograms (**c**)—comparison of Sup (**d**)—comparison of MED views (R-Sup and L-Sup); (R-Med and L-Med). "Retraction" phenomenon in the left breast with a hypoechoic central area (*arrow*) which corresponds to the tumor. The tumor topography coincides in projection with the X-ray mammogram data. In the right breast, both X-ray mammogram and ABVS show the ductal ectasia in the nipple and areola area (*open arrow*)

ABVS tomography techniques. The tumor is surrounded by a hyperechoic halo and desmoplastic reaction manifested by streaking, which should be visible in three mutually perpendicular views: coronal, axial, and sagittal. All nodular masses with this sign in three perpendicular views are proven to be malignant (Fig. 4.33).

Remember that masses without the "spiculation" sign are not always benign. For example, medullary carcinoma constitutes about 1–5 % of all breast carcinomas. This type of cancer has no desmoplasia effect, i.e., no formation of fibrous tissue around the tumor. In noninvasive lobular carcinoma, this feature can also be absent in half of the cases [52]. This feature needs further study on a wider sample of patients with noninvasive types of cancer.

4.4.2   Carcinoma with Microcalcification

Ductal carcinoma is the most common histological type of cancer, occurring in 70–80 % of cases. Its course is more favorable and the growth is less aggressive than in other histological types of breast cancer. One of the earliest manifestations of DCIS mammographically is the appearance of pleomorphic clustered microcalcifications [53]. A relatively reliable sign of malignancy is the presence of 15 calcifications per 1 cm^2 of breast tissue [54]. Microcalcifications are usually located in the central area of the tumor replacing the destroyed cancer cells and in the lumen of the ducts. The more microcalcifications are found in a limited area, the higher the risk of malignancy. Grouped microcalcifications are often found in patients with a low number of estrogen receptors in breast tumors. The detection of microcalcifications is of particular importance when the tumor contour cannot be confidently delineated. Microcalcifications are always clearly visible in mammography. Therefore, mammography is the leading method for detection of preinvasive tumor types. Ultrasonography and MRI have limited value in assessing microcalcifications.

High-frequency US with the use of 15–18 MHz transducers allows visualization of the microcalcifications, even if sized less than a millimeter (approx. 0.3 mm in diameter). ABVS uses a transducer with a 14 MHz average scan frequency, which also allows identification of microcalcifications sized 0.5–1 mm. They are clearly visible in the 3D stratified analysis of views as bright dots on the background of the hypoechoic nodule. The high sensitivity of the probes used in the ABVS technology enables visualization of a greater number of microcalcifications than in the ordinary mode with multiplanar reconstruction or in cine loop mode (Fig. 4.34).

Breast cancer occurred in relatively young women averaging 41 years in age. About 7–8.8 % of all cancer cases are found in young patients [55]. In this age group, the course of breast cancer is most aggressive and has a poorer prognosis [56]. This finding is in keeping with the literature which shows that more than half of women between 25 and 49 years of age have dense breasts with higher cancer risks, as do approximately 29 % of women older than 50 years [57, 58]. Cancer in young women can look like a benign lesion. The tumor contour should be carefully assessed. A malignant tumor almost always has irregular contours. Sometimes it is jagged or with a small undulation of the edges of the nodule. Therefore, when sonographically examining young women with an oval-shaped lobulated mass with somewhat indistinct margins, one should remember that a similar pattern can be observed also in triple-negative cancer. We have a similar case in a young woman, 38-years-old, with the long-term follow-up of a benign breast mass (Fig. 4.35). Follow-up US showed a lobulated mass without distal shadowing, weakly vascularized, measured 1.0*0.5 cm, resembling a fibroadenoma. Mammography was performed a year ago. It showed the presence of dense glandular tissue, with isolated microcalcifications in the upper-inner quadrant of the left breast. The patient was followed by physicians with a US exam every 6 months. The mass increased in size slightly, fine-needle aspiration biopsy was performed, and no cancer cells were found. The mass was finally considered a fibroadenoma. One year later, mammography was repeated. The images in both views showed

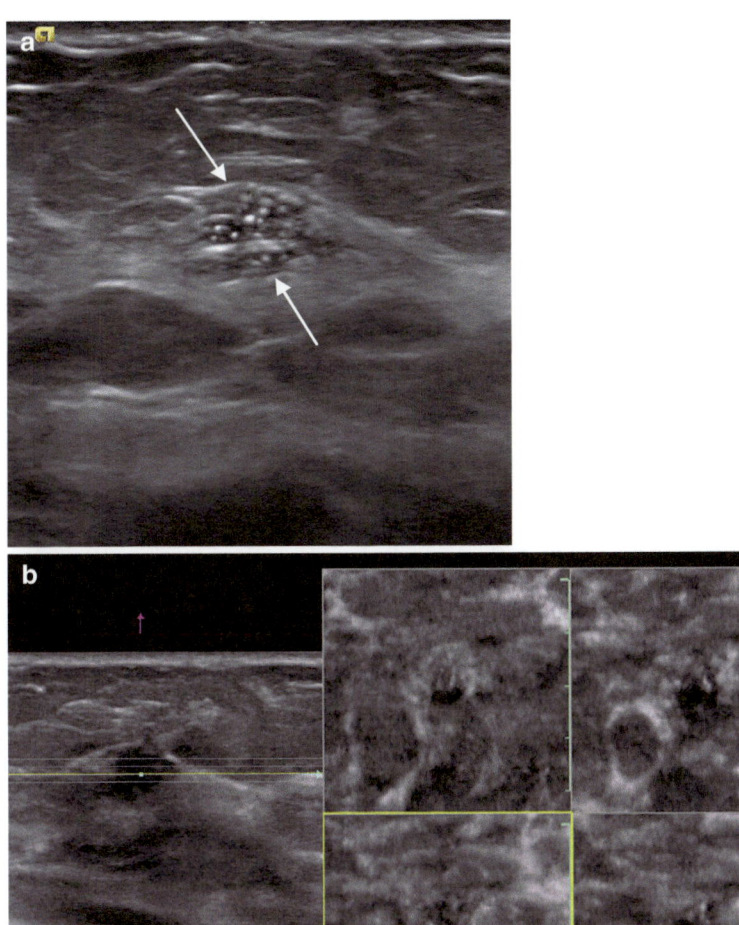

Fig. 4.34 Nonpalpable invasive ductal carcinoma of a 62-year-old woman, T2N0M0, luminal type B, G2 grade. Comparison of HHUS and ABVS. (**a**) The small-sized tumor 4*6 mm is present as clustered microcalcifications visible on HHUS. (**b**) ABVS tomogram. Combination of multiplanar and multislice views. On the coronal slices obtained through the tumor, microcalcifications can also be detected

pleomorphic microcalcifications clustered in the border of the dense glandular tissue. The mass in the left breast was considered as BI-RADS 5—high probability of malignancy. An ABVS tomogram was indicated for precise topography. On the ABVS, signs of malignancy were also revealed. The 3D US study also clearly identified microcalcifications in the mass. A moderate "retraction" phenomenon stellate appearance and a distortion of the lesion contours were clearly defined around the hypoechoic lobulated nodule. After exact topographic examination, sectoral resection was performed. The tumor was diagnosed as invasive ductal carcinoma about 2 cm in diameter, triple negative type.

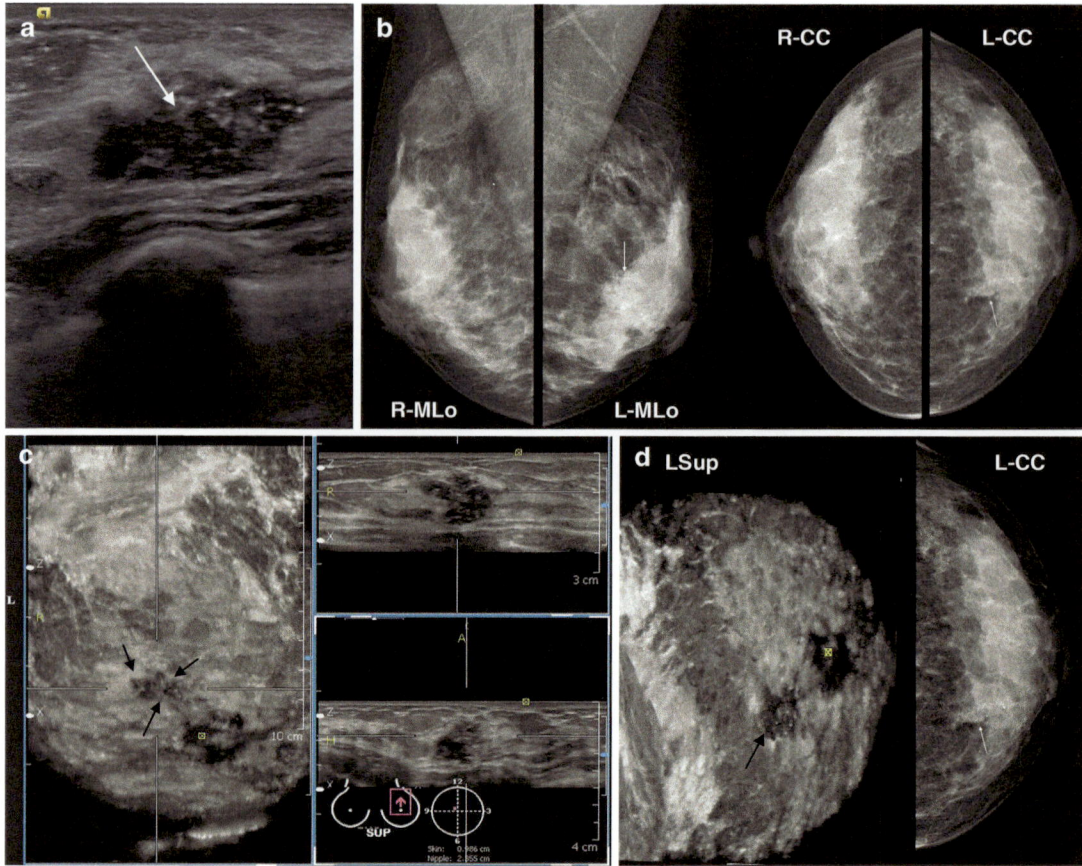

Fig. 4.35 A palpable mass in a 38-year-old nulliparous woman in the upper-inner quadrant of the left breast. Histopathology confirmed invasive ductal carcinoma, T2N0M0, TN type, grade G2. Comparison of HHUS, MMG, and ABVS. (**a**) HHUS. A hypoechoic mass 20*8 mm with irregular contours, with microcalcifications was classified as BIRADS 3 initially. (**b**) Bilateral side-by-side comparative mammograms. Comparison of symmetrical views (R-MLo and L-MLo, R-CC and L-CC). The tumor remains occult on the MMG, only an area of glandular distortion and asymmetry is noticeable in the left breast (*white arrows*). A slight asymmetry with accompanying pleomorphic microcalcifications is seen in the deep areas of the left breast. (**c**) ABVS tomograms. Image analysis using an ABVS workstation. Multiplanar reconstruction (sagittal typical view—on the *top right part*; coronal view—*left part*; axial—on the *bottom right part*). Detection of the tumor's topography (*arrows*) in three perpendicular views. The ABVS image shows a good tissue contrast between the tumor and glandular tissue itself with demonstration of a stellate pattern. (**d**) Side-by-side comparison of the ABVS tomogram (*left part*) and MMG (*right part*) in similar views. The benefits of ABVS in visualization of a tumor in dense breasts are obvious

4.4.3   Lobular Breast Carcinoma

Lobular carcinoma constitutes 5–15 % of all diagnosed breast cancers, differing from intraductal carcinoma by a less favorable prognosis and more aggressive course [52, 59, 60]. According to a recent epidemiological study, the incidence of lobular breast cancer is increasing, especially among postmenopausal women. The likely cause of this increase is thought to be the use of complete hormone replacement therapy [61]. Because the ILC is difficult to diagnose mammographically, higher false-negative results have been reported for ILC than for IDC patients [62]. This is because ILC is manifested by the process of microcalcification much more rarely than DCIS and this type is characterized by the formation of less dense lesions compared to those in IDC [63]. ILC are also difficult to diagnose clinically because they often appear as diffuse infiltrative processes with no clinically palpable masses [64]. ILC has a tendency to spread diffusely or between the collagen fibers of the breast and produces little desmoplastic response [62]. Sonographic detection of ILC may be difficult too; the sensitivity for lesions smaller than 1 cm is between 25 and 85.7 % [65–68]. Usually the most common sonographic appearance is a hypoechoic, heterogeneous mass with irregular or indistinct margins and posterior acoustic shadowing [54]. In addition, ovoid types of ILC predominate with smooth but indistinct margins which can also appear as benign masses [52]. Therefore, mammography and HHUS often provide equivocal data.

Small-sized lobular cancers are very rare. In most cases, the tumor is surrounded by a hyperechoic halo with a slight "streaking" phenomenon. The described case was diagnosed originally by HHUS during the interval period before mammography screening. The tumor measured 5×4 mm. It was a round hypoechoic lesion with irregular margins and a hyperechoic halo which was easily detected despite the small size. Unscheduled mammography also confirmed the occurrence of a 5 mm mass, which was not visualized a year ago (Fig. 4.36). Such a small tumor required preoperative US guidance marking. To clarify the topography of the mass for tumor resection, an ABVS study was performed. The tumor was located in the axillary process 9 cm from the nipple. Histological examination confirmed the diagnosis of lobular carcinoma in situ.

ILC is associated with a higher rate of multiplicity and bilaterality [60]. In most cases, the multiplicity is false as the slice contains the same tumor growing along a convoluted duct. If a multicentric tumor is suspected, the mammographic study can sometimes be completed by MRI. ABVS also allows determination of the type of tumor growth providing a global breast image. An integrated approach to ABVS ultrasound simplifies the search for multifocal and multicentric tumors. ABVS tomography detects suspicious areas with the high-density effect, and ABVS reveals the "retraction" effect that helps search for additional tumor nodes on the whole-breast tomographic images.

This can be illustrated by a case of multifocal invasive lobular cancer in a woman with a previous history of breast surgery due to fibroadenoma 20 years ago. The tumor developed in the same breast close to the resection line, which was clearly shown by ABVS. An HHUS study was performed after a screening mammogram due to increased breast density and scattered fibroglandular breast parenchyma. HHUS showed two subtle lesions in the left breast with blurred margins, which looked benign at first sight. Due to the small size, both nodules demonstrate no vascular supply on a Doppler mode but showed increased stiffness in elastography mode, not typical for benign changes, and therefore required further investigation. It was decided to perform an ABVS tomogram to characterize the nodes. The whole volume was analyzed in the coronal plane moving slowly from the nipple level down to the chest wall. A previous resection line or scar deformity was clearly seen in the lower-inner quadrant of the left breast, despite the surgery being a long time ago. Very close to it, the largest node was clearly visible on the ABVS tomogram in all views, with a stellate appearance and with a minimum "retraction" pattern. And the smaller nodule was also visible due to the typical "stellate" pattern also in the lower-inner quadrant. ABVS tomograms were resliced in the sagittal and axial planes, using magnification, in order to find additional lesions. No additional lesions were seen in the coronal plane. Quadrantectomy was performed after wire localization of the tumors. The multifocality of the tumor growth was confirmed by histopathology (Fig. 4.37).

The sign of architectural distortion in the area of a growing tumor is much more serious and more characteristic of ILC [69, 70]. It is observed in approximately 10 % of represented cases [60]. The histological growth pattern of ILC does not have a tendency to form a mass [71]. However, the asymmetry can be a structural option for a normal gland, as well as a result of dyshormonal hyperplasia. The usual radial direction of fiber elements from the gland base to the areola is disrupted, the harmony of the matrix is lost, unusual shadows with streaks appear, and trabeculae are thickened [59]. Architectural distortion of

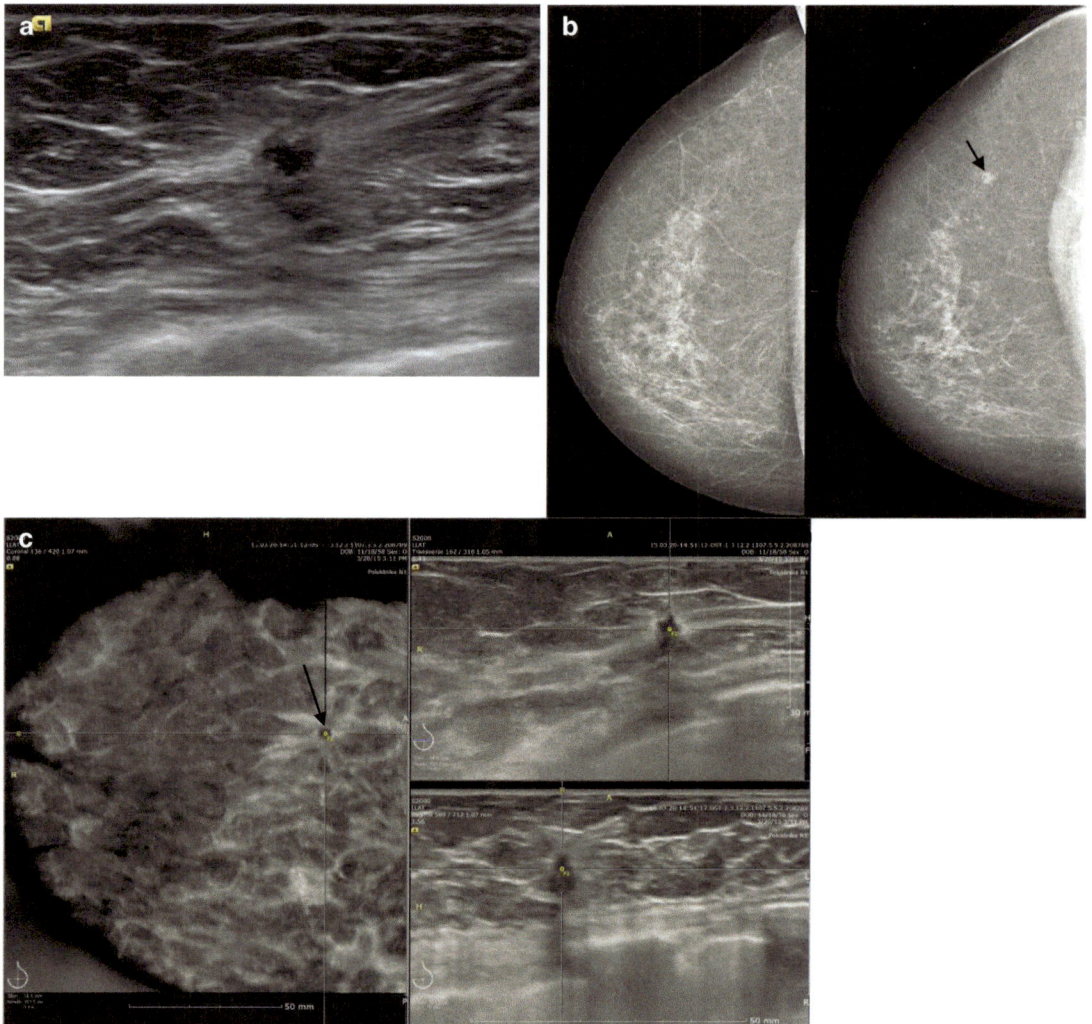

Fig. 4.36 Interval cancer in a 67-year-old woman which was present as a nonpalpable mass on a screening HHUS. LCIS (lobular carcinoma in situ), T1aN0M0, grade G1. HHUS, ABVS, and MMG performance. (**a**) A small-sized 4*5 mm hypoechoic mass with irregular contours and a hyperechoic halo is seen within residual breast fibrosis tissue. (**b**) Follow-up MMG in the similar CC projections of the left* breast (screening MMG—*left part*, MMG performed 9 months later—*right part*). (* X-ray mammograms are rotated on a horizontal axis to allow better visual comparison with ABVS). A small nodule with relatively low density appears on a follow-up MMG in less than 1 year (*arrows*). (**c**) ABVS. Image analysis on the ABVS workstation shows the tumor's topography in multiplanar view. The tumor is located in the axillary process and has a pronounced "retraction" pattern, exceeding the dimensions of the nodule itself, despite its small size and the absence of signs of tissue invasion the tumor is seen on the ABVS quite evidently. The *yellow circle* marks the location of the nodule

the normal parenchyma is obvious compared to that in neighboring unaffected areas on bilateral mammograms. Bilateral breast structural analysis in conventional HHUS is absolutely impossible. Therefore, an ABVS tomogram can help to identify infiltrative type of cancer growth due to the global breast assessment and possibility to make side-by-side comparisons of

breast architecture on the ABVS workstation. A review of the coronal images may be helpful for distinguishing between real lesions and nonhomogeneous areas [72].

In the following case, conventional HHUS failed to show the tumor itself, and mammography depicted the structural abnormality in the deep lower part of the left breast and measured it

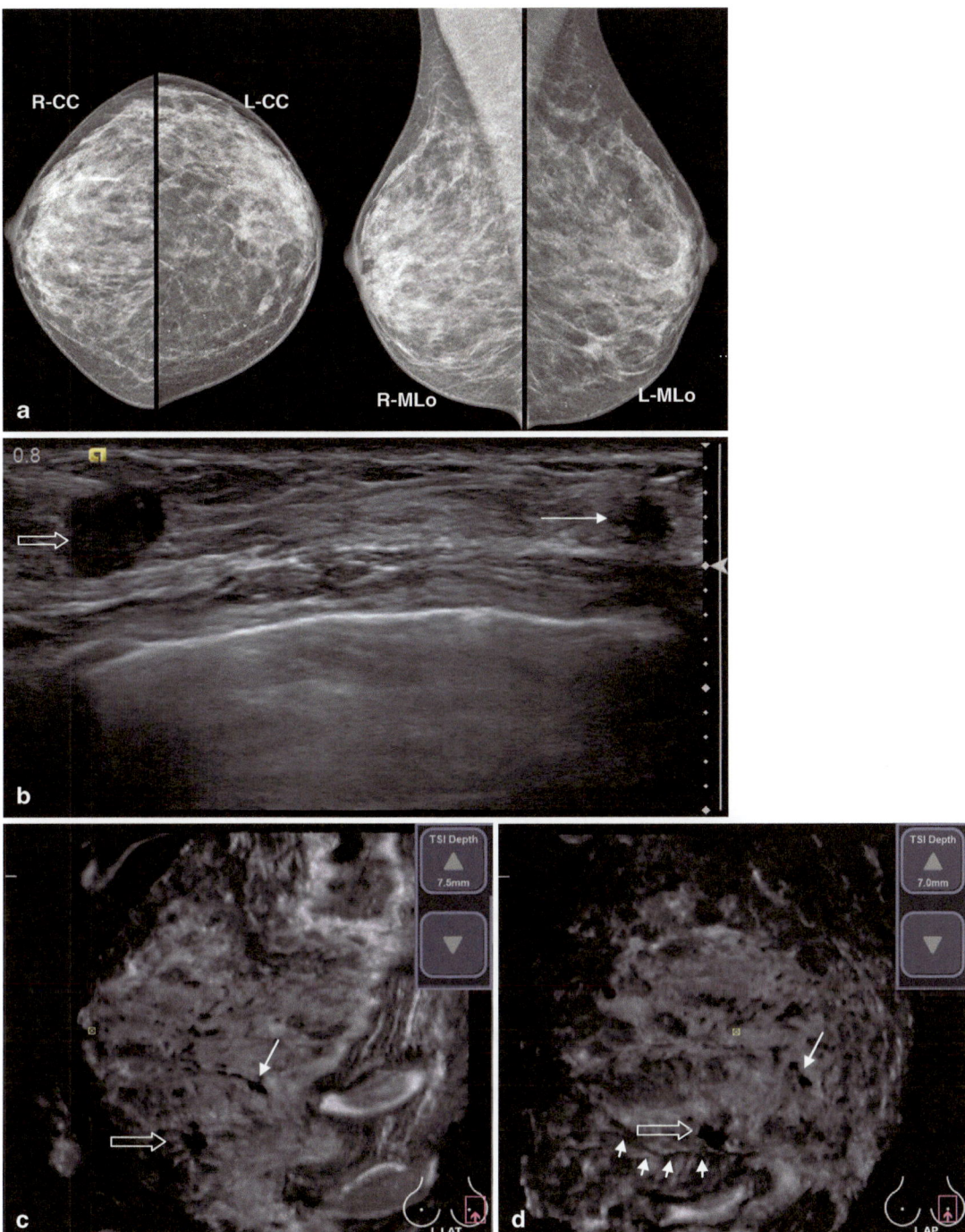

Fig. 4.37 Multifocal breast cancer in a 48-year-old woman, ILC, 2T1N0M0, luminal type A, grade G1. Comparison of HHUS, ABVS, MMG. (**a**) Bilateral side-by-side comparative mammograms in CC and MLo views (R-MLo and L-MLo, R-CC and L-CC). No clear evidence of any suspicious nodule in the dense breast. Scattered fibroglandular breast parenchyma. (**b**) Two hypoechoic nodes with indistinct boundaries and increased anteroposterior size, the first 8 mm (*open arrow*) and the second

4 mm (*single arrow*), are visible on HHUS. (**c, d**) ABVS shows two lesions in the lower quadrant with polycyclic contours and mild "retraction" effect. (**c**) L LAT view—latero-medial oblique view of the left breast. (**d**) L AP view—left anteroposterior coronal view. In the inner-lower quadrant of the left gland, a scar deformity is visible (*short arrows*) lying close to the nodule (*open arrow*) with an irregular shape. The second nodule, which is very subtle, is also seen on the coronal view (*long white arrow*)

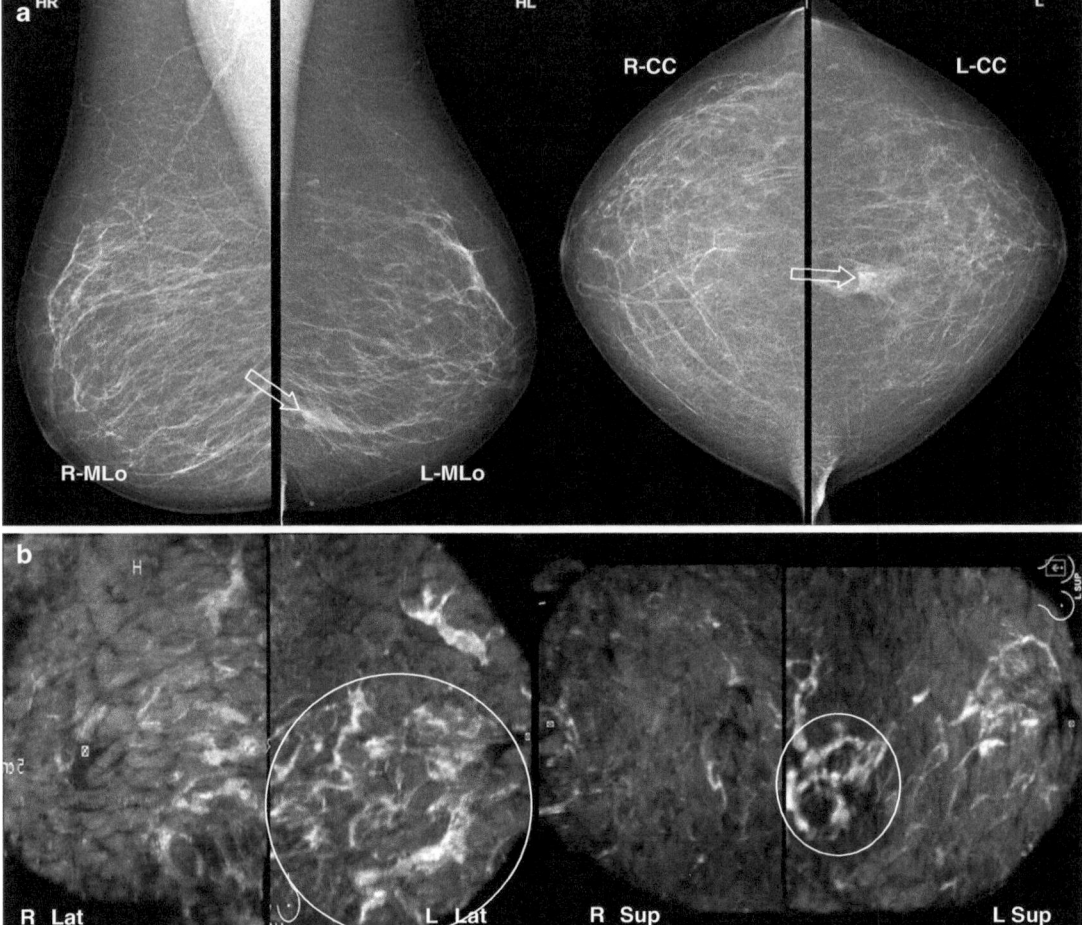

Fig. 4.38 Invasive lobular carcinoma in a 62-year-old female. T3aN0M0, luminal type B, grade G2. Comparison of MMG and ABVS data. (**a**) Bilateral side-by-side comparative mammograms in CC and MLo views (R-MLo and L-MLo, R-CC and L-CC). Area of structural deformity with streaks is seen in the left breast (*open arrows*). (**b**) Bilateral side-by-side comparative ABVS tomograms in Sup and Lat views. An asymmetry and structural distortion are also seen on the ABVS images. Streaking is noted on the border of the lower quadrants (*white circle*). The dimensions of this area are significantly larger than those on the X-ray mammogram. Pathomorphological size of the removed tumor was close to that shown on ABVS

as 2.5 × 1.5 cm, while an ABVS tomogram found architectural distortion in the same region with increased echogenicity in a larger area, measuring up to 3.5 cm in diameter (Fig. 4.38). Histopathology defined the size of the tumor nodule as similar to that determined by ABVS (3.5 × 2.5 × 1.5 cm). This can be explained by lack of compression during the ABVS study, which results in precise tumor measurement. Thus, the ABVS tomogram was superior to MMG in estimation of the tumor volume in cases of infiltrative growth of lobular cancer.

4.4.4   Cancer in Women with Dense Breast

Breast cancer is so multifaceted that its manifestations in the mammogram and sonogram are covered in numerous works. Some cancers are not visible on a mammogram, and they are called occult or negative, and some are difficult to find using US. Dense breast tissue has been proven to be the most important inherent limitation of MMG in the diagnosis of breast cancer as some cancers are missed, often requiring ultrasound to complete the breast imaging assessment [57]. In addition, dense fibroglandular tissue is associated with increased risk of breast cancer and also lowers the sensitivity of MMG to as low as 30–48 % [9, 48, 73, 74]. Cancers detected in women with dense glandular background are usually larger, less differentiated, and more often with metastasis in lymph nodes. Cancer in dense breast tissue is 18 times more often identified within a year after negative mammographic screening [9, 48].

According to our data, the ABVS technique is a valuable supplement to mammography in dense fibroglandular tissue. Our data are consistent with those of other researchers who also consider ultrasound as an alternative method of cancer detection at early stages in dense breasts, due to better contrast of the hypoechoic tumor against the hyperechoic fibroglandular breast tissue [46]. These are the abovementioned cases of small tumors not exceeding 1–2 cm in women with dense breasts in whom US was superior to MMG in evaluation (Figs. 4.31, 4.35, and 4.37).

Breast cancer in women with dense breast is more likely to be diagnosed later, at the stage of axillary lymph node metastasis. All the following cases are dedicated to occult breast cancers, when the tumors were clearly defined in their true sizes only by ABVS performed after negative data of mammogram and controversial result of HHUS. These tumors were measured at more than 7 cm (!) in the first case and more than 10 cm (!) in the second case. In the first case, a 42-year-old woman presented with a self-identified painful breast mass. Inflammation was suspected on conventional HHUS initially because the patient was rather young and had a symptomatic breast. Sonographically a hypoechoic 2.5*5.5 cm region was found in the right breast with increased blood flow, with right axillary lymphadenopathy also typical for inflammation. All these features were characteristic also for mastitis or fibrocystic mastopathy with inflammatory changes. The diagnosis of breast cancer was not suspected initially. Further evaluation with mammography showed equivocal data. Bilateral side-by-side comparison of craniocaudal and mediolateral oblique views showed tightened glandular tissue, especially in the upper-external quadrant in the right

breast at a considerable distance, and scattered microcalcifications in all quadrants. Fine-needle aspiration biopsy failed to identify cancer cells. Anti-inflammatory therapy didn't give relief. An ABVS tomogram was performed 2 weeks after the HHUS and MMG. The large centrally located infiltrative lesion appeared on coronal ABVS slices with a desmoplastic reaction and streaks into the outer and lower quadrants. The whole tumor measured 6*7*2.5 cm (Fig. 4.39).

In the second case, in a 60-year-old woman, mammography screening did not reveal any changes in the dense breasts with pronounced fibrocystic mastopathy of 6 months earlier. An HHUS exam was performed due to a noticeable breast asymmetry, and in the right breast lump, large hypoechoic masses were seen. The repeated mammogram showed a zone with increased density on the border of the upper quadrants with indistinct margins measuring 5 cm at the longest and an enlarged axillary lymph node in the right breast. An ABVS tomogram particularly clearly visualized the replacement of the glandular tissue in the right breast by a tumor 12*10*2 cm, occupying the whole breast (Fig. 4.40). The large ABVS probe provides whole coverage and characterization of the large mass. During the follow-up study of those two cases after neoadjuvant chemotherapy, ABVS might provide an accurate measurement of the tumors as they are larger than 5 cm.

All presented cases demonstrate the benefits of an integrated approach in cancer detection using X-ray mammography, HHUS, and ABVS in cases of increased breast density.

4.4.5 Cancer in Breasts with Fat Involution

On the contrary, when there is no distinct contrast between the tumor and fat tissue, the possibilities of US are inferior in detection of structural changes in early tumor stages. Therefore, mammography is the principal technique in fat involution, being much more sensitive compared to US. Identification of masses with ABVS in women with fatty involution has

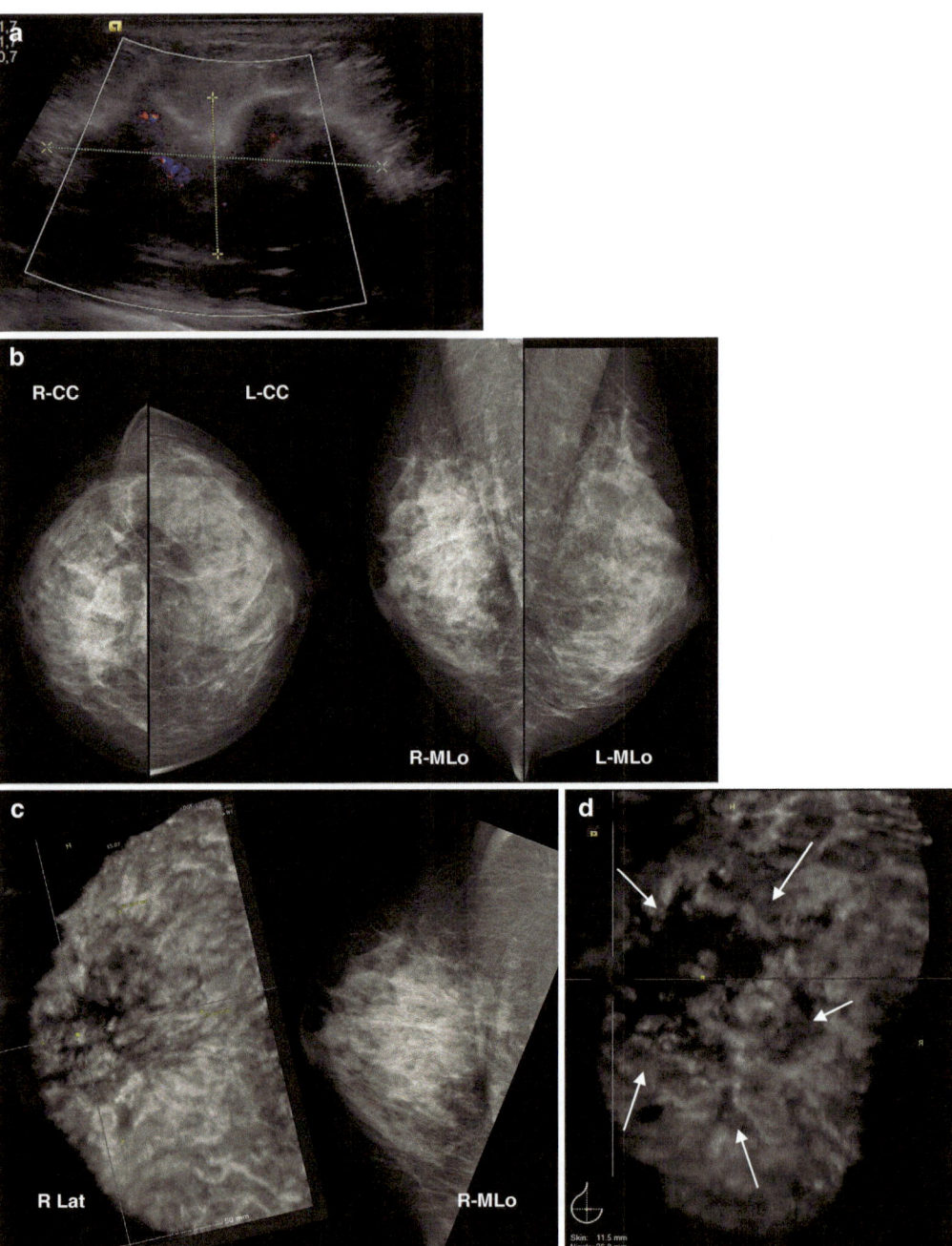

Fig. 4.39 Mammographically occult breast cancer manifested as mastitis in a 42-year-old patient. IDC, T3aN1M0, luminal type A, grade G2. Comparison of HHUS, MMG, and ABVS. (**a**) HHUS in Color Doppler mode. Hypoechoic shadow-like region measured 5*2 cm with irregular contours and severe distal shadowing showed chaotic color signals inside. (**b**) Bilateral side-by-side comparative mammograms in CC and MLo views (R-MLo and L-MLo, R-CC and L-CC). Dense breasts with a slightly enriched glandular structure in the central area of the right breast. Significant breast density is mimicking tumor infiltration. (**c**) Side-by-side comparison of ABVS and MMG in corresponding views of the breasts (ABVS* R Lat view—*right part* and MMG MLo view—*left part*). *ABVS image is rotated counterclockwise for better appreciation of comparison. On ABVS, a large centrally located tumor is seen. On the mammogram, the tumor itself is not clearly distinguished from the dense fibrous breast tissue. (**d**) Image analysis of the tumor (*arrows*) on an ABVS workstation. A hypoechoic tumor lies centrally. The nipple area is marked by a *rectangle*

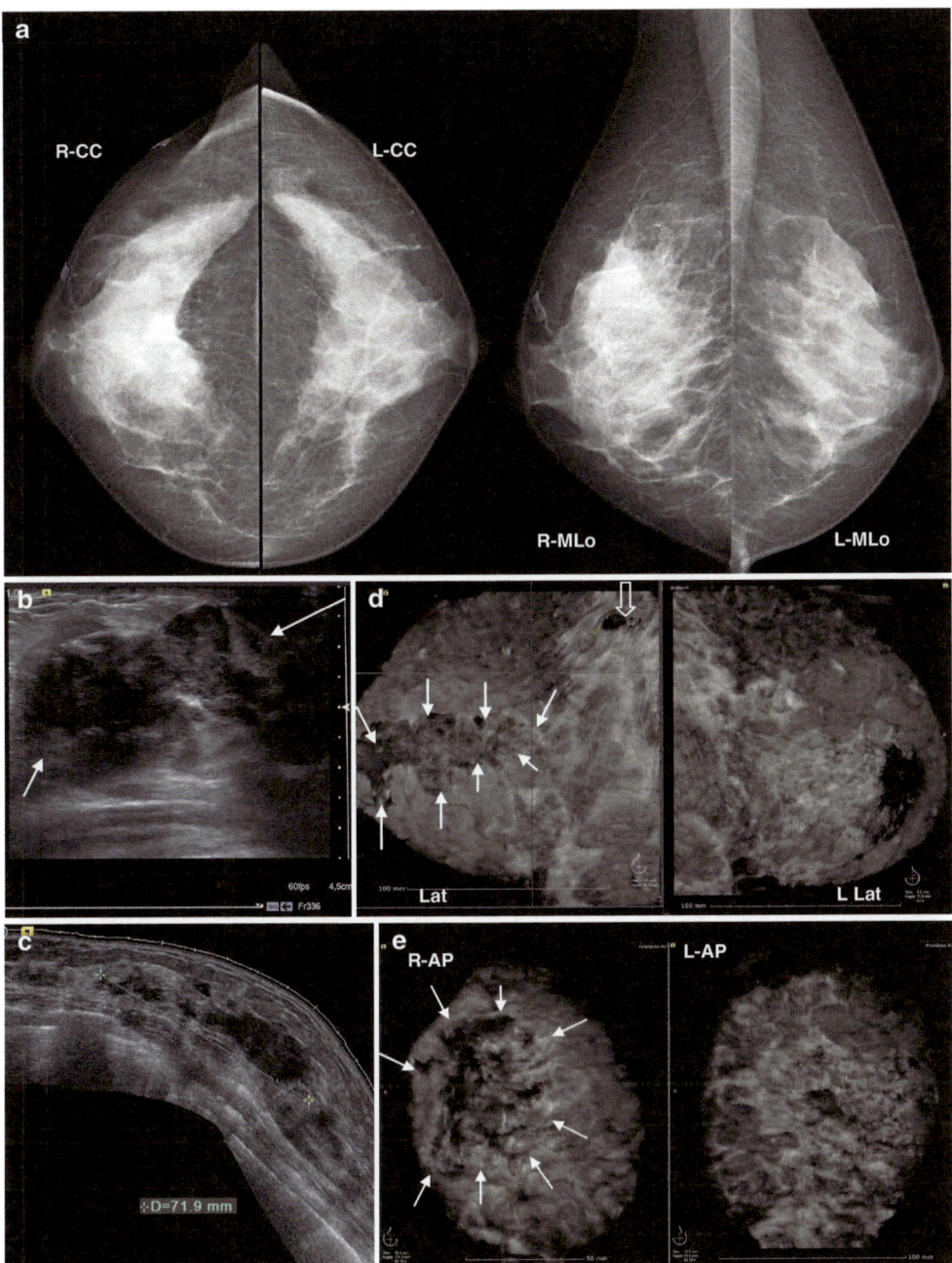

Fig. 4.40 Mammographically occult cancer in dense breast in a 60-year-old patient with a positive axillary lymph nodule. IDC of the right breast, T3aN1M0, luminal type A, G2 grade. (**a**) Bilateral side-by-side comparative mammograms in CC and MLo views (R-MLo and L-MLo, R-CC and L-CC). Significantly dense breast masking the tumor. (**b**) On HHUS, a hypoechoic mass with indistinct contours with difficulties in displaying the whole tumor in 1 FOV (field of view) with conventional linear probe. (**c**) Conventional HHUS when using Siescape panoramic imaging enables better tumor measurement. The longitudi- nal size of the tumor is 7 cm. (**d**) Side-by-side comparison of the ABVS tomograms on the workstation. Bilateral com- parison of latero-medial oblique views (R Lat, L Lat). ABVS shows tumor occupying all central regions and extending deeper through the breast (*arrows*). The sentinel nodule is seen in the axillaries region, ensuring the diagno- sis (*open arrow*). (**e**) Side-by-side comparison of ABVS tomograms on the workstation. Bilateral comparison of anteroposterior views (R AP, L AP). In the left breast, the central regions are represented by glandular tissue. In the right breast, the tumor replaces the glandular tissue (*arrows*)

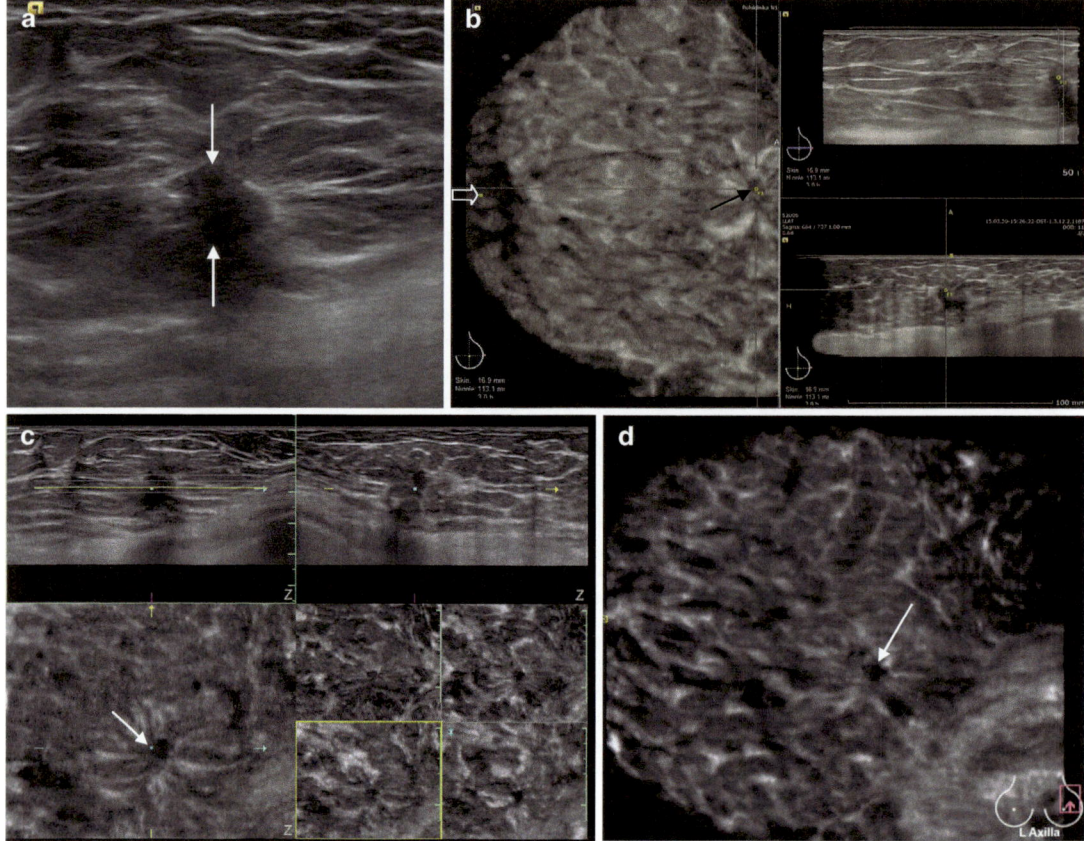

Fig. 4.41 A case of cancer in a fatty involute breast in a 52-year-old woman. IDC, T1N1M0, luminal type B, G2 grade. Comparison of HHUS and ABVS data. (**a**) HHUS. A hypoechoic nodule on a background of adipose tissue with moderate distal shadow is seen (*white arrows*). (**b**) Analysis of the L Lat ABVS view on a workstation. Multiplanar reconstruction through the tumor nodule in the left breast. A hypoechoic nodule with retraction effect (*white arrow*) is seen in the marginal area 12 cm from the nipple (*open arrow*). (**c**) Analysis of the tumor on an ABVS device. Combination of multiplanar and multislice reconstruction modes. "Retraction" phenomenon is visible around the tumor in coronal views. (**d**) ABVS. Axillary view. Tumor (*arrow*) has echogenicity lower than that of fat tissue. It is surrounded by a radiant crown

its own features; the parenchymal symmetry should be carefully analyzed.

This should be taken into account in ABVS studies due to the obscure shadow masses in patients with fat involution. The identified X-ray findings should be topographically compared with the ABVS tomograms obtained to reveal the true pattern of the mass (Fig. 4.41).

Basal-like tumors have interestingly been shown to exhibit epithelial-mesenchymal transition, a feature of aggressive tumors, and these may relate to MMG and sonographic morphology of these tumors (less spiculation) relating to high tumor grade and poor prognosis. Histological characterization of BRCA 1 tumors (basal) has demonstrated that many of these tumors demonstrate a pushing margin. This is a feature of medullary tumors. A pushing margin refers to tumor cells not separated by connective tissue. This has been shown to correlate with a smooth nonspiculated mass on mammography and the lack of an echogenic halo on US [75]. Spiculation is not a characteristic sign of invasive tumors but often accompanies them. In a noninvasive tumor, spiculation is not a characteristic sign. Thus, the presence of other symptoms such as irregular margins, hypervascularity, increased stiffness, and absence of a hyperechoic rim is of value in suspecting malignancy (Fig.4.42).

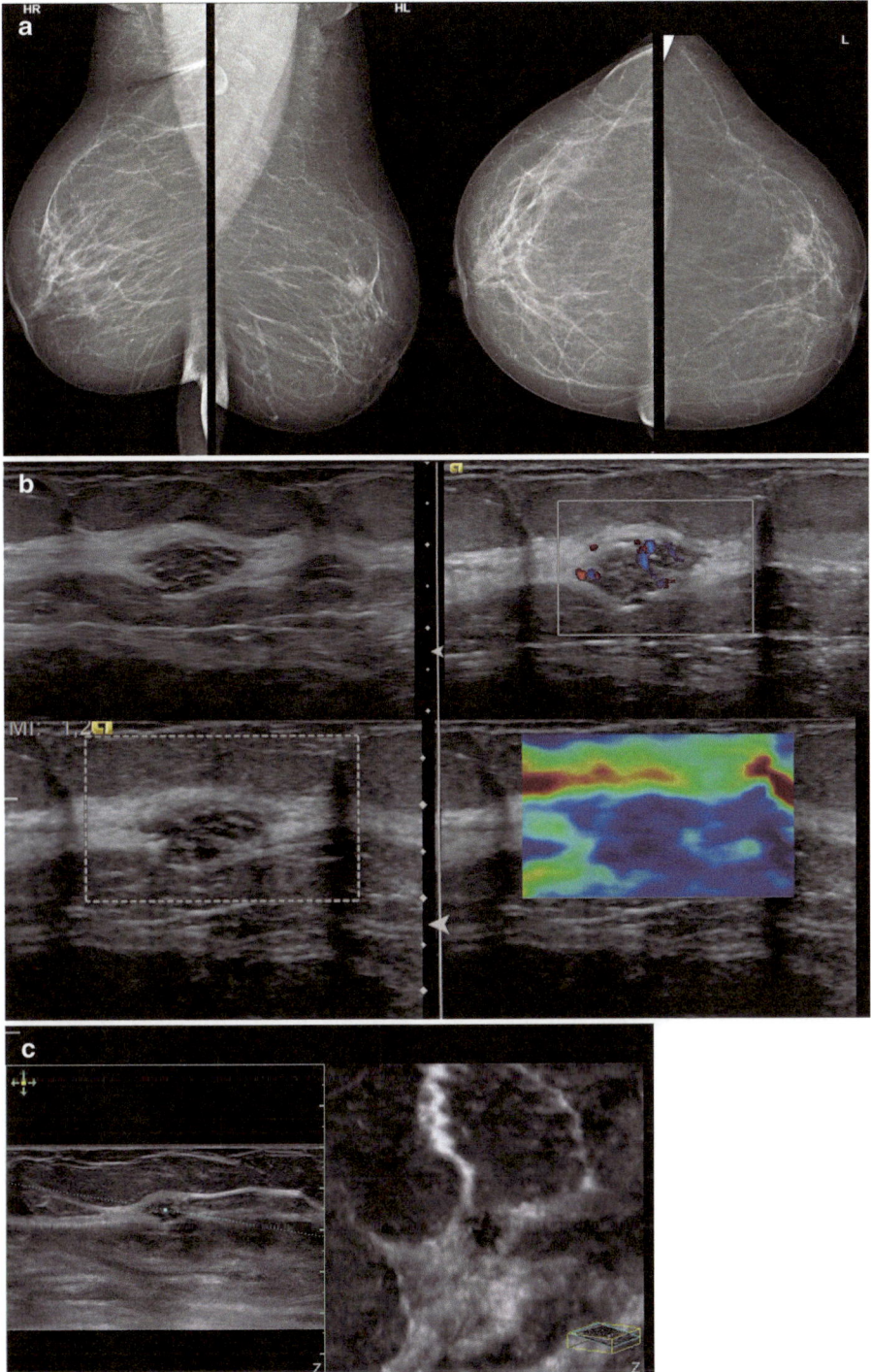

Fig. 4.42 A case of LCIS in a 60-year-old woman. Comparison of HHUS with Color Doppler and elastography, MMG, and ABVS data. (**a**) Bilateral side-by-side comparative mammograms find a subtle lesion in the left breast. (**b**) Multiparamentric HHUS shows an isoechoic tumor on B-mode without clear signs of malignancy, simi-lar to the locally fatty lobule (*left part*) in Color Doppler mode (*top of the image*), elastography mode shows an increased stiffness in the lesion (*bottom of the image*). (**c**) ABVS images obtained through the tumor. Coronal slices of the lesion demonstrate no "retraction" phenomenon, but uncircumscribed margins and stellate pattern

4.4.6   Multifocal and Multicentric Breast Cancer

Multiplicity of tumor nodules equally occurs both in lobular and in ductal carcinoma [76–79]. As mentioned previously, lobular carcinoma has a high tendency to multifocal growth. The frequency of multifocal foci occurrence does not depend on the molecular or histological type of the tumor. It is important to identify all the foci as in a multifocal lesion the surgery volume is always decided in favor of organ removal or quadrant or lumpectomy instead of tumor resection. Therefore, before the surgery, any suspicious foci should be identified.

The frequency of additional cancer detection increases with the size of the primary tumor. So, if the primary node is >2 cm, additional microinvasive foci spreading into the surrounding breast tissue at a distance of 4 cm are histologically verified in 28–60 % of cases [79]. The definition of therapeutic tactics and prognosis for breast cancer depends largely on the stage of the disease, which is also directly linked to the size of the primary lesion. For foci exceeding 2 cm, a 5-year survival rate is not achieved by eight out of ten women. For tumors sized up to 1 cm, 92 % of patients survive for 20 years without relapse [76, 77].

Tumor size evaluation by palpation is definitely subjective and depends on the experience of the examiner. The shape and consistency of the tumor is closely connected to its histological type. Scirrhous tumors are significantly more stiff, and their dimensions by palpation exceed the size of the tumor estimated by X-ray and HHUS. Medullary tumors have a softer consistency, and their size by palpation is generally consistent with that determined by X-ray and ultrasound.

Unfortunately, both mammography and HHUS do not always yield tumor dimensions and outline their margins accurately. Half of T1-stage tumors are overestimated by mammography, and HHUS failed in assessment of the margins of shadow-type tumors. If multiple lesions are suspected, it is recommended to perform MRI-mammography with contrast enhancement [78, 80]. Ultrasound also allows the identification of additional tumors. But, unfortunately, the aperture of the standard US transducer is only 4–6 cm, and it cannot cover the whole gland or large tumors exceeding 5 cm. To avoid these disadvantages, an ABVS tomogram with a 16 cm transducer scanning field is suggested, allowing the global evaluation of the breast (Fig. 4.43). With the help of ABVS, exact localization of three invasive lesions in order to get an idea of the required resection volume was performed. The superior and inferior limits of the area were clearly identified. This was of value for surgical planning of sectorectomy for an acceptable cosmetic result. The histological results revealed clear resection margins for all three lesions.

ABVS also allows precise measurement of a tumor, even a shadow-type tumor, in multislice and multiplanar modes (Fig. 4.44). The slice thickness can be set minimally as 0.5 mm or 1 mm, and tumors can be visualized in coronal planes in order to evaluate the maximum tumor size and its depth.

4.4.7   Locally Advanced Breast Cancer

Among all the cases of verified breast cancer, about 20 % are of a locally advanced type. These include cancers measured over 5 cm with lymph node invasion and nipple, skin, or chest fascia invasion, as well as cancer of any size with conglomerated lymph nodes. The leading technique for the diagnosis of locally advanced cancer forms is MRI with contrast enhancement, mammography, and ultrasound which are inferior, except for cases of a tumor spreading anteriorly toward the skin and nipple [80, 81].

A tumor growing in the surface layers of the gland appears on a mammogram with a lymphangitis track extending from the edge of the tumor to the skin. It causes local tissue restructuring, roughness of the internal contour of the skin strip, thickening of the skin, and its retraction (the so-called "button" sign). In the subareolar zone, the "cancer bridge" sign is apparent, that is the deformation and nipple retraction when it is involved in the lesion [9]. The altered thickness of the skin, the disappearance of the contour of

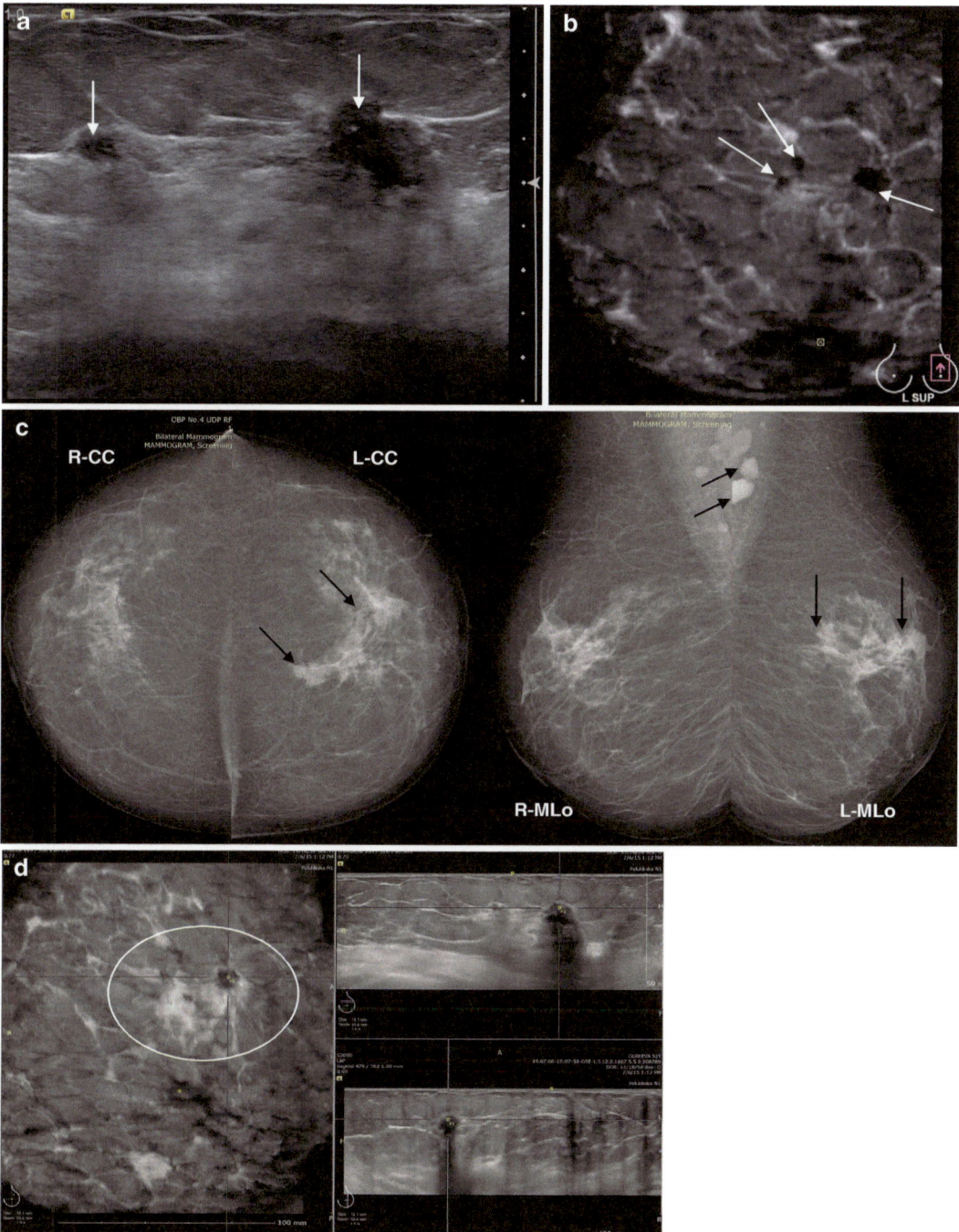

Fig. 4.43 A case of multifocal breast cancer in a 64-year-old woman. T3bN3M0, luminal type B, grade G2. Comparison of HHUS, MMG, and ABVS data. (**a**) HHUS shows only two hypoechoic nodules with distal shadow and irregular margins (*arrows*). (**b**) ABVS. L Sup view (left superior-to-inferior direct view). Three hypoechoic nodules with spiculation are seen in one projection (*arrows*). (**c**) Bilateral side-by-side comparative mammograms in CC and MLo views (R-MLo and L-MLo, R-CC and L-CC). Multiple tumors are seen in the left breast with retraction (*black arrows*). Positive lymph nodes in the left axillary region. (**d**) ABVS. Workstation processing of anteroposterior coronal slices of the left breast. Multiplanar reconstruction mode through the largest nodule. The area of structural deformity is visible in the identified area (*circle*). ABVS tomogram shows o'clock topography of the structural changes, which is seen on the pictogram

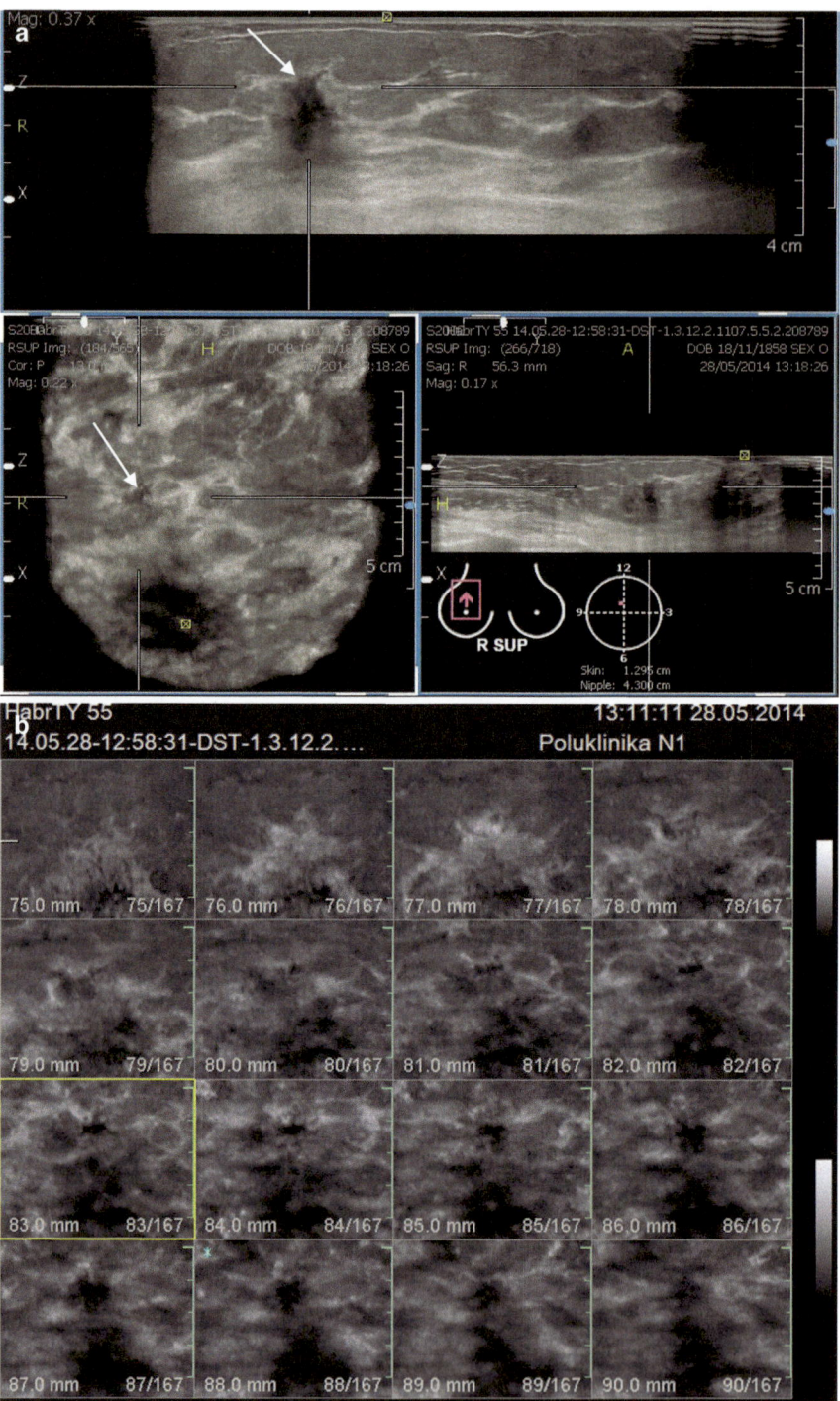

Fig. 4.44 An example of image analysis of breast cancer on an ABVS unit and on a workstation. Patient X., 55-year-old. T1N1M0, IDC, G2 grade, luminal type B. (**a**) Image analysis on an ABVS workstation. Multiplanar view through the tumor in R Sup projection (superior-to-inferior view). Typical longitudinal view (*top of the image*), *left bottom*—coronal view, *right bottom*—axial view. Determination of the topography of the mass. The hypoechoic lesion with retraction lies in the upper-outer quadrant of the right breast (*arrow*). (**b**) Multislice reconstruction on the ABVS unit through the tumor. Slice thickness is 1 mm. The tumor is not yet visible in the first images, but a radiant crown is visualized around it when the slices go deeper

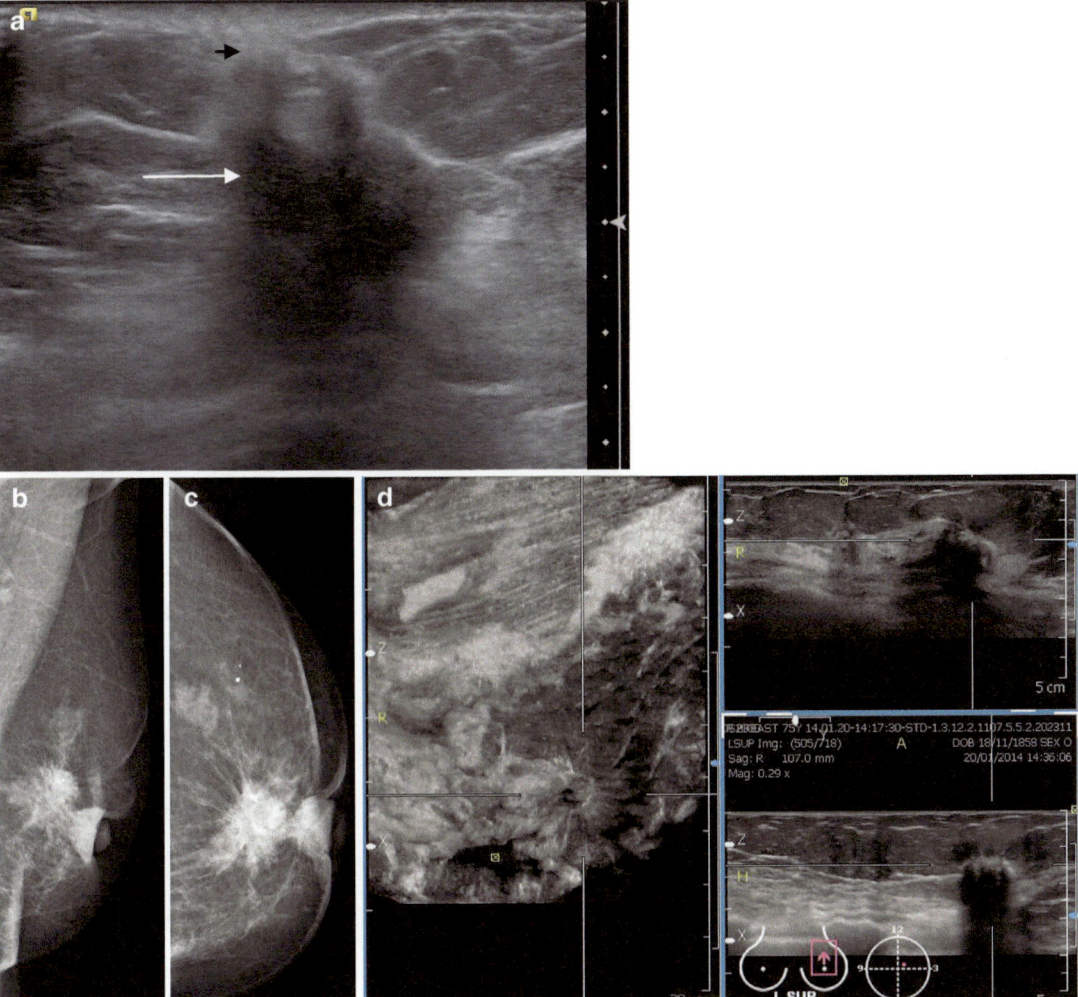

Fig. 4.45 A case of IDC with nipple invasion in a 70-year-old woman. T4N1M0, G2, luminal type B. Comparison of the performance of HHUS, MMG, and ABVS. (**a**) HHUS. Tumor with severe posterior acoustic shadowing (*white arrow*) with projections into the premammary fat tissue and invasion into the skin (*black arrow*). The thickening of the skin at the site of invasion is clearly visible, without a border between tumor and derma. (**b, c**) X-ray mammograms. (**b**) MLo view. C) CC view. The disappearance of a hypoechoic subareolar area. The nipple is tightened to the tumor. (**d**) ABVS. Image analysis on a workstation. Multiplanar view through the tumor. Determination of the topography of the mass. The tumor is located above the nipple and displaces it downward

premammary fat, the clear involvement of the nipple, and the disappearance of a hypoechoic subareolar zone can also be seen in ABVS tomograms if the tumor invades the derma of the nipple (Fig. 4.45).

In deep centrally localized tumors, involvement of the thoracic fascia and underlying chest muscles should always be suspected. When the tumor is fixed to the chest wall, which can also be detected by palpation, a mammogram can show the roughness of the contour of the deep layer of the superficial fascia, and if the tumor invades toward the pectoralis muscle, the mammogram shows the opacity of the adjacent region of the fat tissue. If the tumor is shadow type and located at the base of the gland, conventional ultrasound can form a false impression of the presence of tumor spread on the pectoral muscles. Macromastia can

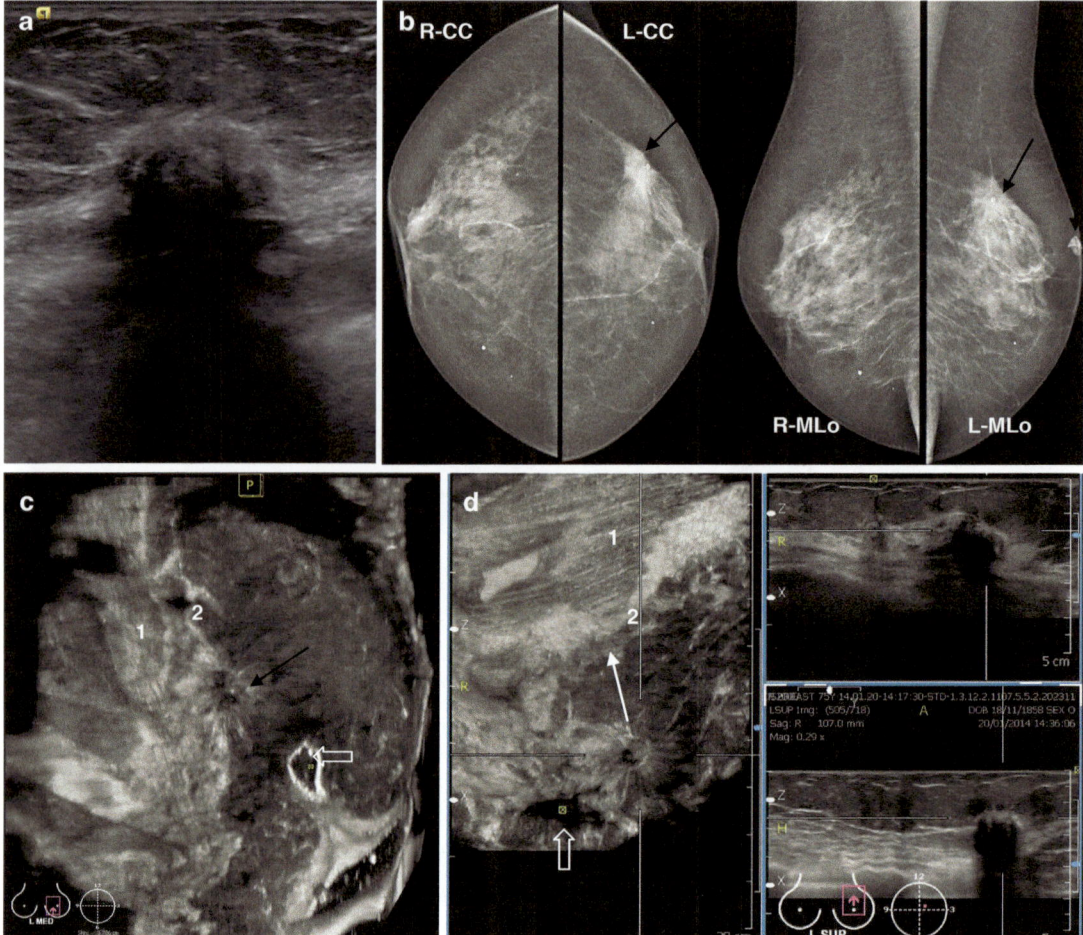

Fig. 4.46 An example of a shading type of breast cancer which simulates fascial invasion. IDC of the left breast, T2N0M0, G2 grade, luminal type B. (**a**) HHUS. Tumor with severe distal shadowing. The massive distal US-shadow precludes the clear visualization of the invasion of the tumor in the breast muscles. (**b**) Bilateral side-by-side comparative mammograms. R-CC, L-CC, R-MLo, and L-MLo projections. Retraction of the nipple of the left breast and strands from the tumor to the nipple are visible. The tumor is visible as a large solitary node with an expressed streaking. (**c**) ABVS. Image analysis on the workstation. L-Med view (oblique mediolateral view of the left breast). Tumor invasion into the superficial pectoral fascia is suspected. The tumor is located on the thoracic fascia (*2*), and the tumor crown is superimposed on the image of the pectoral muscles (*1*). The nipple is retracted (*open arrow*). (**d**) ABVS. Multiplanar reconstruction mode through the tumor. Analysis of the frontal upper slice of the left breast. The tumor is displaced with the gland when changing position, which is clearly visible by the shifting of the tumor from the fascia and pectoral muscles (*bidirectional arrow*)

mask the posterior contour of even non-shadow tumors. To solve this problem, an ABVS tomogram can be used in the "mammographic" views. A change of the patient's body position causes the tumor's displacement, and the distance from the tumor to the chest wall increases. To clarify the integrity of the fascia's contour, it is worth using multislice mode or two view modes, adjusting the shear line on the deepest regions of the tumor facing the retromammary area. If there is no invasion into the muscular layer and the fascia, the linear order of muscle fibers will not be disrupted. The retromammary fat tissue can be seen between the fascia and the tumor, indicating the absence of invasion (Fig. 4.46).

Treatment of locally advanced cancer is a complicated and controversial process that involves a combination of chemotherapy, immunotherapy, hormone replacement therapy, surgery, and radiation therapy. This complex approach to breast cancer treatment causes primary inoperable patients to be candidates for surgery after treatment. The assessment of the spread and size of the tumor becomes particularly relevant in this case to follow up the lesion. Mammography is certainly a reliable method of assessing the size of the tumor, but follow-up studies of tumor response to chemotherapy are performed preferably with an ultrasound study and even better with an ABVS tomogram that allows accurate and objective determination of the lesion development.

4.4.8 Primary Multiple Breast Cancer

Bilateral breast lesions are detected in 0.8–19.6 % of cases. This variability can be explained by the use of different diagnostic modalities for the detection of bilateral primary multiple breast cancer, as well as by different approaches to the criteria for its primary character [79].

Cancer development of both breasts that is simultaneous or separated in time by no more than 3–12 months is called synchronous cancer. Breast cancer development in both breasts within a time interval from 2 to 29 years is called metachronous cancer. The third form of primary multiple breast cancer is metastatic, with changes in the second breast occurring within 5 years after surgery. The frequency of metastasis is 9.9 % [79]. When examining patients with BI-RADS 5 tumors, the contralateral breast should also be carefully examined in all views. The stored digital information will help in identification of synchronous and metachronous cancer.

4.4.9 Difficulties in Identifying Some Cancer Localizations

Some areas are not completely displayed on a mammogram. In the craniocaudal view, these are the upper-deep region of the breast, and in the oblique view, it is the deep-medial region

of the breast and the deep-lateral part of the gland. On ABVS, the upper quadrants can be seen better due to features of the positioning, and this view can complement the mammography data. The most illustrative in this regard are examples of tumors located in the upper-deep region of the breast and not visible in the craniocaudal view (Fig. 4.47). The dense glandular tissue also obscures visualization of the tumor in the oblique mediolateral view. However, the upper-inner quadrant on the anterior view fully covers the area of the tumor and demonstrates the characteristic radiance. Lesions in the upper-deep region of the gland can be seen using the possibilities of the ABVS tomogram.

Many researchers noted the limitations of the ABVS technique in the examination of the axillaris regions [81, 82]. This reduces the possibility of using the method in screening. One of the known manifestations of breast cancer on a sonogram is an increased or changed axillary lymph node; also cancer can be found in the axillary breast processes or accessory breasts located in this area. A number of works recommend an additional scan of axillae in the 2D mode or in an automatic mode if cancer is suspected from the ABVS data [81]. This is possible in patients with significantly developed fatty tissue; however, in lean patients, this study can't be performed without artifacts and the emergence of "no-show" areas. In cases when the lesions are significantly remote from the contour of the gland (axillary process, accessory lobe), an additional scan of this area is needed, if the patient's body composition allows. On the anterior and oblique views, the tumor of the axillary area is placed out of the scanning field and can be omitted. The standard examination scheme can be used: 2D ultrasound with US angiography, ABVS tomography, and visual inspection of the axillary areas. To avoid these false-negative cases, one can perform mammograms and conventional ultrasound. If this order is changed, cancer of an axillary process can be missed as in the case below where the ABVS tomogram was carried out without prior mammography and limited to the standard ABVS tomogram positions, so the axillary area was not

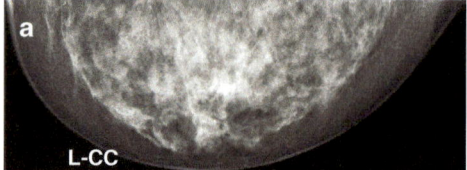

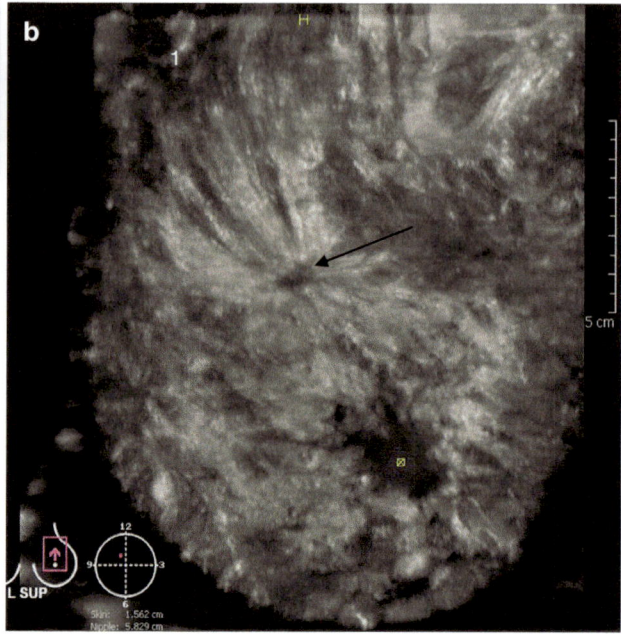

Fig. 4.47 IDC of the left breast, in a 50-year-old patient, T1aN0M0, G1 grade, TN type. Comparative multidisciplinary study. (**a**) X-ray mammogram. Craniocaudal view, direct view (L-CC). The tumor is not visible in a frontal image due to its location in the upper-posterior region of the gland. The only note is the streaking from the upper contour of the gland to the nipple. (**b**) ABVS. L Sup slice (left superior-to inferior view). The tumor is clearly visible with significant "retraction" phenomenon

fully displayed (Fig. 4.48). A direct mammogram in the craniocaudal view also did not reveal the tumor, because it is located in the deep-outer region in the area of axillary process, but multiple masses are clearly visible as a chain in the axillary area in the oblique mediolateral view on the mammogram. Retrospective analysis of the saved ABVS tomogram data allowed visualization of only part of the tumor located at the top of the breast, and another two masses (overlying) did not enter the field of view.

4.5   Male Breast

The normal male breast is composed of adipose tissue, several ducts, and a number of stromal elements. Kupffer ligaments are not expressed in the male breast. The development of glandular lobules in men occurs from increased sensitivity of the breast tissue to normal circulating estrogen levels [83]. Gynecomastia is a frequent condition in men of various ages; it is detected in 36 % of healthy young men and in 57 % of healthy older men on physical examination and more than 70 % of hospitalized elderly men [84]. Physiological gynecomastia occurs during neonatal and pubertal periods. Pathological gynecomastia affects older men and has multifactorial causes. Obesity is one of the most common causes of hyperestrogenicity in men due to increased peripheral aromatization of androgens. The risk of male breast cancer development in men with gynecomastia and a body mass index >30 is doubled [84]. Chronic illness also promotes increased production and decreased utilization of estrogens resulting in gynecomastia [85]. Gynecomastia manifests as a palpable firm mass. It was considered that 30–70 % of male breast cancer occurs on the basis of gynecomastia. Male breast cancer accounts for approximately 1 % of all cases of cancer in developed countries [86].

As with breast cancer in women, the standard diagnostic approach is clinical examination, followed by mammography and biopsy. With 92 %

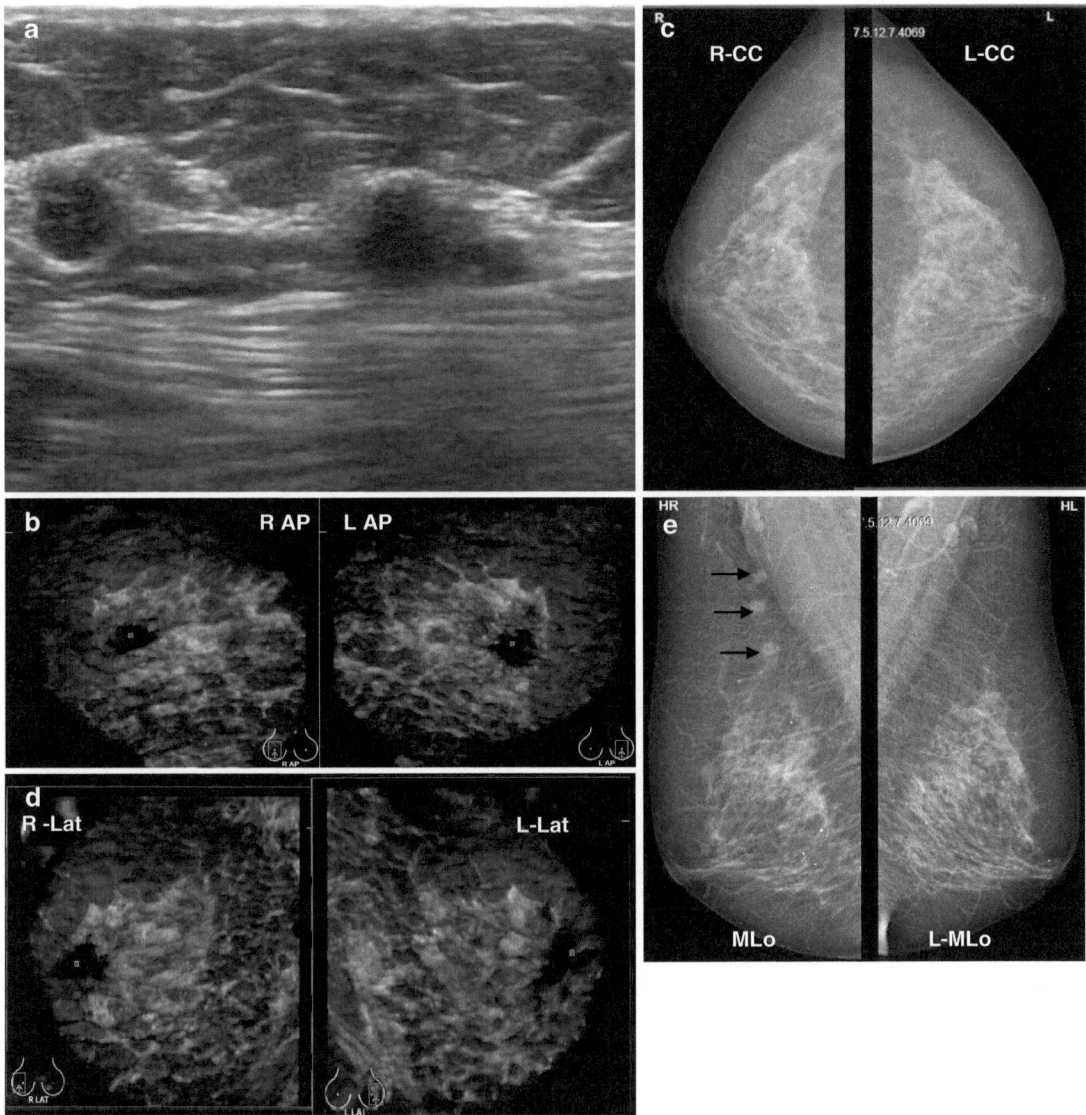

Fig. 4.48 Multifocal IDC in the axillary process in a 63-year-old woman, 3T1N0M0, G2 grade, luminal type B. Performance of the different visualization modalities. (**a**) HHUS. Several hypoechoic tumors with indistinct boundaries. (**b**) ABVS. Bilateral anteroposterior coronal views. The symmetry of the image with a predominance of the glandular component in the internal quadrants. (**c**) X-ray mammogram. Bilateral craniocaudal images (R-CC and L-CC). Tumors are not visible in the right gland on the frontal view. (**d**) ABVS. Bilateral latero-medial oblique views. In the glandular triangle area, the tumors are also not identified. (**c**) X ray mammogram. Bilateral MLo views. Multiple nodes with dense indistinct boundaries in axillary process (*arrows*)

sensitivity and 90% specificity [87, 88], MRI is used in the diagnosis of advanced cancer [89]. Ultrasonography is reported as a method of choice with quite good sensitivity in evaluation of gynecomastia and diagnosis of male breast cancer [90].

4.5.1 Adiposomastia

Pseudogynecomastia or lipomastia (fatty breast), which is most common in obese men, must be distinguished from true gynecomastia. It is excessive fat deposition without the presence of ductal structures in the breast tissue [91]. The primary technique in differentiation of lipomastia from gynecomastia is mammography. Mammography shows only the transparent adipose tissue in the structure of the breast, without any inclusions and streaking. US shows no echogenic tissue behind the nipple. An ABVS tomogram shows no discoid shaped layer of echogenic glandular tissue behind the nipple on a coronal slice (Fig. 4.49).

4.5.2 Gynecomastia

In true gynecomastia, there is firm discrete sub-areolar tissue or diffuse fibroglandular tissue that resembles a female breast [92]. Gynecomastia is a relatively common breast lesion in men. It should be distinguished from lipomastia. In boys it is caused by dishormonal processes (pubertal gynecomastia) and regresses in several months under the influence of treatment or even without it. In adults (usually older than 45), an increase in breast size is most often secondary and may be caused by various processes: prolonged use of some drugs (such as digitalis and antihypertensives), cirrhosis, chronic kidney disease, prostate cancer, diabetes, and other diseases [93]. Gynecomastia can be unilateral or bilateral. Drug-induced disease will spontaneously resolve after drug withdrawal. Or tamoxifen and local radiation can help to reduce the symptoms. Surgery is the treatment of choice in long-standing disease.

There are three main mammographic appearances of gynecomastia, namely, nodular, dendritic, and diffuse. Nodular gynecomastia appears as a fan-shaped density radiating from the nipple. The MMG appearance of dendritic gynecomastia is a retroareolar soft-tissue density with prominent extensions that radiate into the deeper adipose tissue. Usually it is a feature of long-standing disease. The diffuse type is characterized by heterogeneous dense female breast [94].

An ABVS, tomogram shows clearly nodular type gynecomastia as discoid hyperechoic tissue comprised of glandular tissue that is surrounded

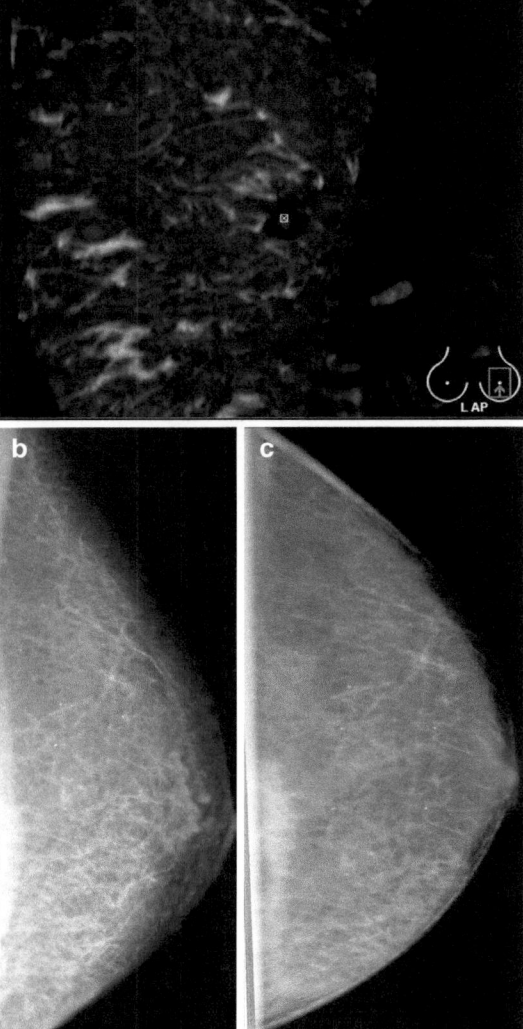

Fig. 4.49 Lipomastia in a 75-year-old male with body mass index more than 30. Comparison of the appearance on ABVS and MMG. (**a**) ABVS tomogram of the left breast in a coronal view (L AP). The breast structure consists of adipose tissue with uniformly lowered echogenicity, and of fibrous septa. (**b, c**) X-ray mammography. MLo—medio-lateral oblique view (**b**); CC—craniocaudal direct view (**c**). Uniform transparency of the breast due to the fat tissue

by hypoechoic fat tissue (Fig. 4.50). ABVS coronal images are most informative for the diagnosis of gynecomastia due to better contrast demonstration between glandular and adipose tissues.

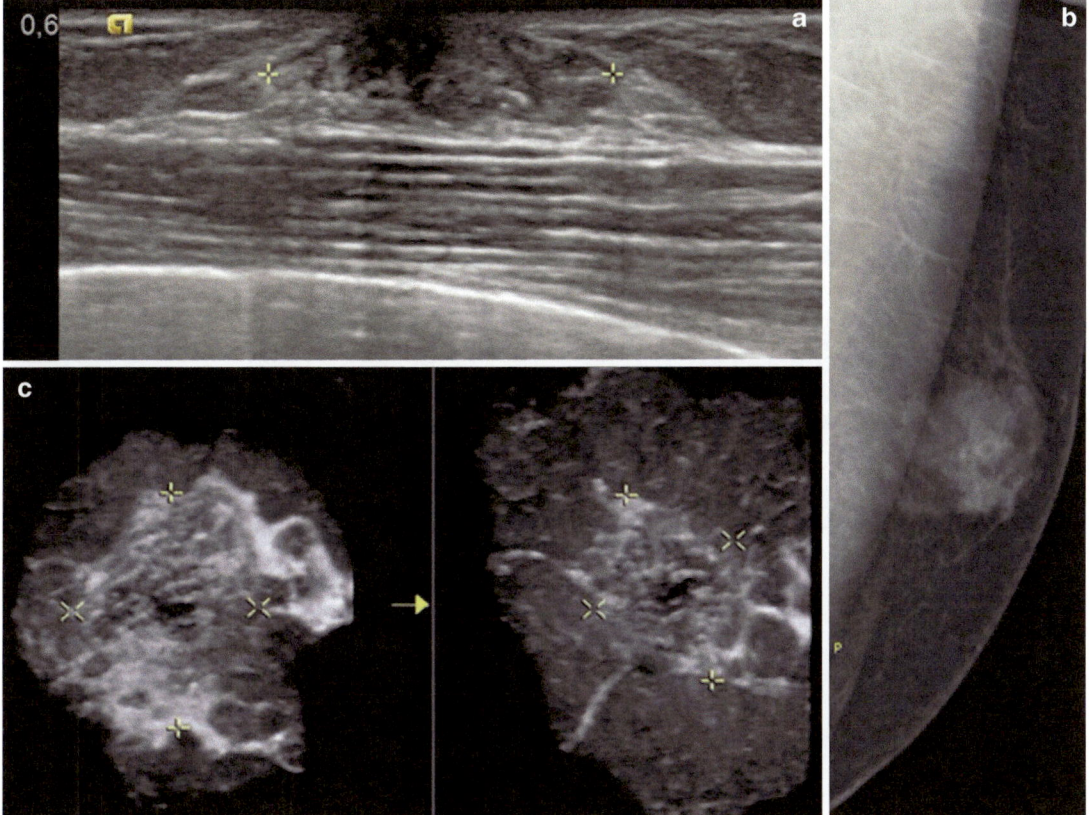

Fig. 4.50 Unilateral left-sided gynecomastia in a 45-year-old male with liver cirrhosis. (**a**) HHUS shows slightly echogenic glandular tissue behind the hypoechoic nipple-areolar zone. (**b**) X-ray mammogram. MLo view of the left breast. Local area of dense nodule behind the nipple is a nodular type of gynecomastia. (**c**) ABVS tomogram. Coronal view of the left breast in gynecomastia. Echogenic glandular tissue is surrounded by low-echogenic adipose tissue. The size of the glandular tissue could be more precisely measured

4.5.3   Male Breast Cancer

The factors in late diagnosis of the disease are likely to be poor knowledge about breast cancer in men and the absence of screening in high-risk men. Some cases of breast cancer occur in men receiving treatment for prostate cancer; the disease also occurs in pituitary prolactinoma, endogenous overproduction of estrogens, and can develop with hypogonadism as the predisposing factor. Several studies have found a high frequency of orchitis history in men with breast cancer [95, 96]. Difficulties of diagnosis of breast cancer in men are associated with the need to perform a differential diagnosis between breast cancer, gynecomastia, abscess, hematoma, lipoma, or other benign diseases [95].

Cancer is often mistaken for gynecomastia and erroneously treated by "pathogenic" androgen hormone therapy, which stimulates a greater growth and metastasis of malignancy. Distant metastases are detected at diagnosis in men more frequently than in women, and the tumor is relatively larger [96].

The mammographic pattern of male breast cancer is the same as in women. The nipple is affected in men more often than in women. Nipple lesion with retraction is usually an early sign occurring in 9 % of cases because even the smallest tumors can connect with the nipple quickly. In male breast cancer, the dense nodule tends to be in the subareolar location but occasionally is eccentric. The margins may be well defined, ill-defined, or speculated. The

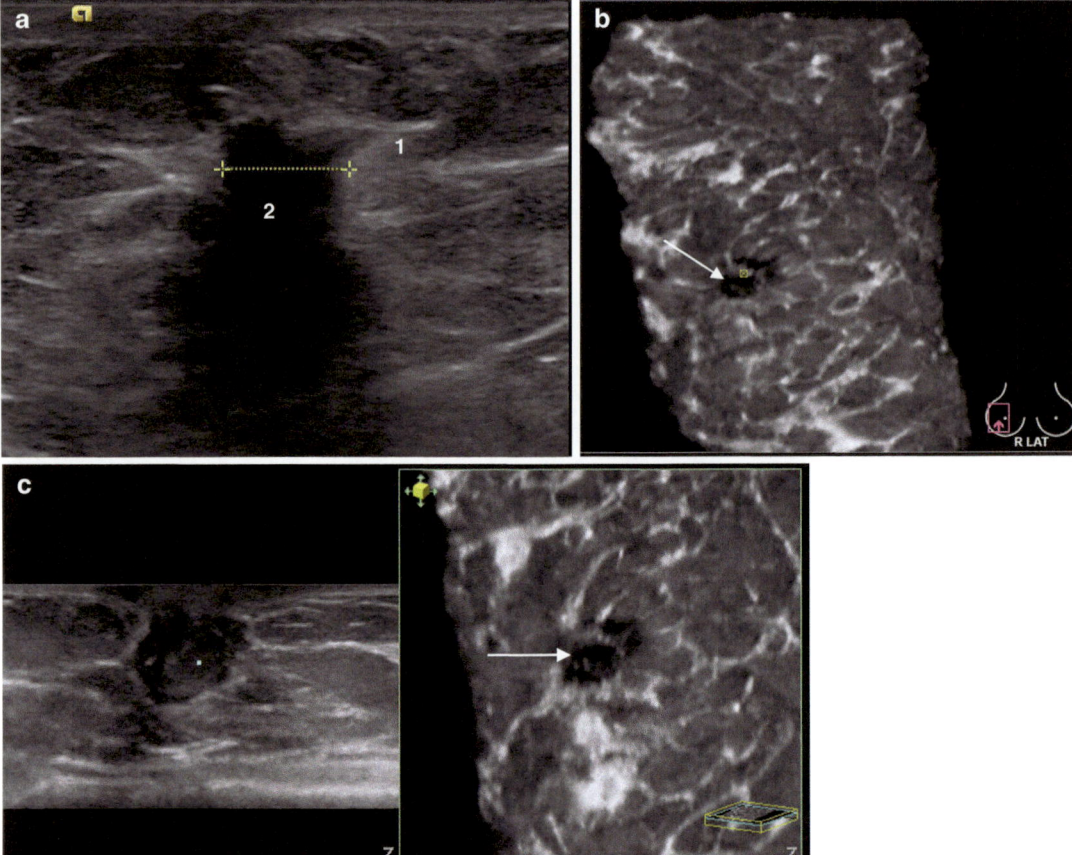

Fig. 4.51 Male breast cancer in a 65-year-old man with gynecomastia in the right breast. Comparison of multimodality approach. (**a**) HHUS. A hypoechoic shadow-type tumor is visualized (*2*) eccentrically from the nipple, surrounded by echogenic glandular tissue (*1*). (**b**) ABVS. Coronal R AP view of the right breast. Eccentrically from the nipple (marked by a *rectangle*), a hypoechoic tumor with "retraction" effect is seen. (**c**) ABVS. Biplanar comparison mode in sagittal view (*left part*) through the tumor provides a coronal slice (*right part*). Spiculated pattern of the tumor nodule is seen (*arrows*)

cancer node is often placed in the subareolar area or more eccentric to the nipple (in contrast to gynecomastia, where the nodular type has a central node location) [97].

Increased mammographic density due to gynecomastia can mimic a tumor. In some cases, the malignant transformation can be suspected by the presence of streaking in the edge of glandular tissue on a mammogram. HHUS fails to differentiate gynecomastia from malignancy [98]. ABVS can distinguish a tumor from gynecomastia (Fig. 4.51). Normally, the nipple in the male breast is represented by a hypoechoic point area. In gynecomastia this area is narrowed. The

principal sign of the presence of a tumor can be an uneven and expanded contour of the nipple-areolar area, with its deformation and displacement from the nipple to the side (Fig. 4.52).

4.6   Mastitis

Mastitis is an inflammatory condition of the breast, which may or may not be accompanied by infection. Mastitis can be associated with lactation, so-called lactational (or postpartum) mastitis and non-lactational, not associated with breastfeeding. Non-lactational mastitis usually

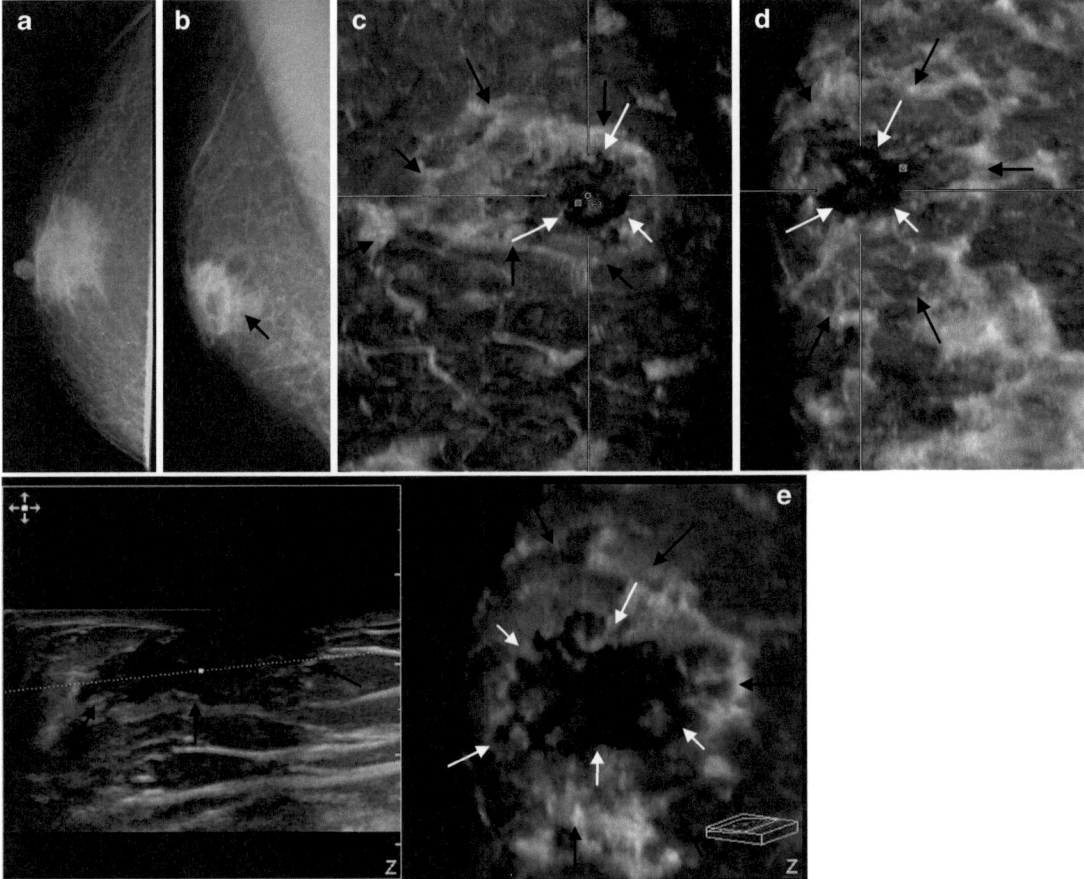

Fig. 4.52 Male breast cancer in a 75-year-old man with gynecomastia after chemotherapy for colon cancer. Comparison of MMG, ABVS. (**a, b**) X-ray mammograms. CC direct view of the right breast (**a**), MLo view (**b**). A dense nodule is visible with a streaky contour eccentrically from the nipple area. The roughness and streaking of the node contour are clearly visible. The tumor is marked by a *black arrow*. (**c–e**) ABVS tomograms. Coronal R AP view (**c**), R Lat view (**d**), biplanar view sagittal (*left part*) through the tumor resulting in a coronal view (*right part*) (**e**). *Black arrows* indicate the contour of glandular tissue. The hypoechoic tumor with streaks (*white arrows*) infiltrating glandular tissue is located inside it

develops due to injuries of the breast or hormonal disorders in women and is a rare condition. Acute mastitis usually develops in the postpartum period. Non-lactational mastitis should be differentiated from inflammatory carcinoma [99–103]. If lactational mastitis is not treated promptly, it will lead to a breast abscess. Breast abscesses are classified according to location: central (periareolar) or peripheral. Peripheral breast abscesses more commonly occur in elderly patients with diabetes mellitus, rheumatoid arthritis, after steroid therapy, recent surgical intervention, or post-radiation therapy [103].

After all, necessary surgical procedures are implemented for treating mastitis, and abscess patients are usually monitored by radiologists. Ultrasound is the first modality, because it is painless, provides guidance for percutaneous drainage if necessary, and can be repeated any time [103]. Ultrasound allows differentiation of the various forms of mastitis in its earliest stages, which is crucial for the selection of the right treatment approach. The quadrants or segments affected by mastitis are of particular interest if surgical intervention is planned. In the early phase, ABVS shows distended ducts, wide

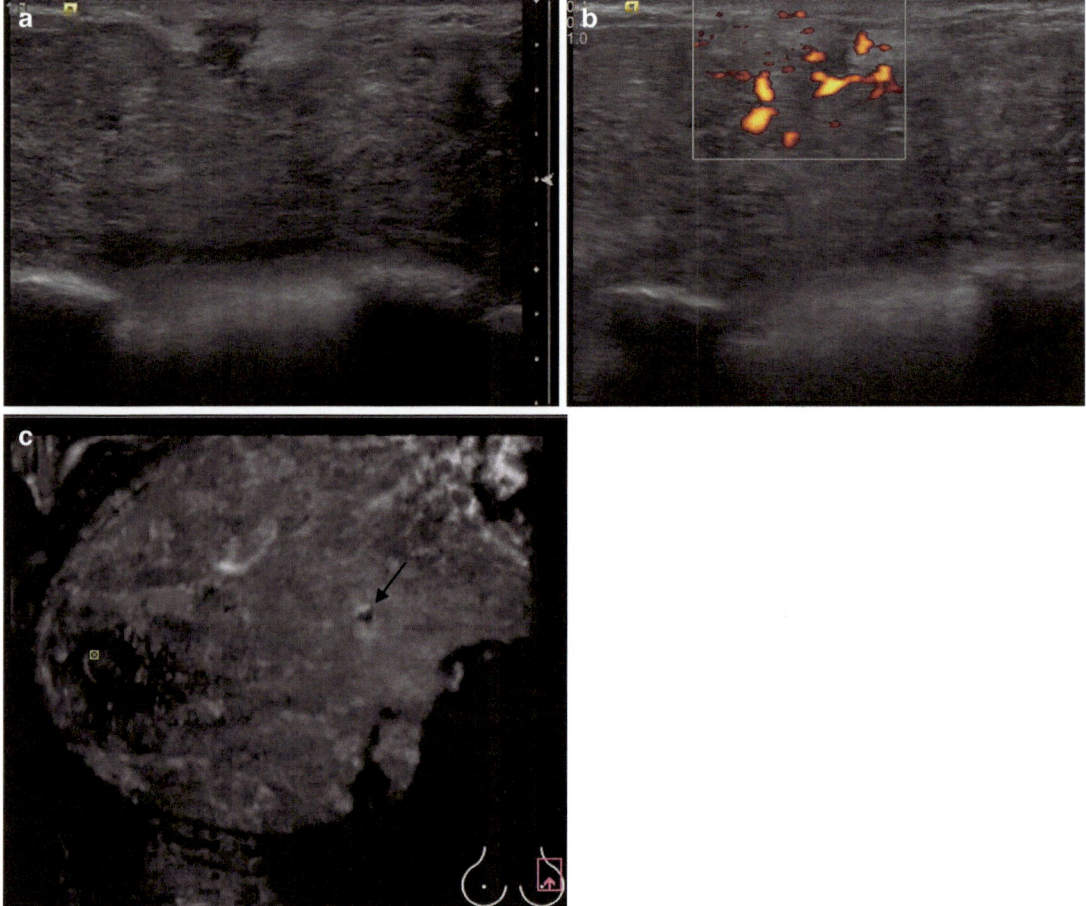

Fig. 4.53 Lactational mastitis in a 25-year-old woman. Comparison of HHUS and ABVS performance. (**a**) HHUS. The breast is uniformly isoechoic, with the superficially located hypoechoic region being inflammatory infiltrate. Linear horizontal stripes indicate the lactiferous ducts. (**b**) HHUS in Power Doppler mode. The presence of increased vascularization around the region. (**c**) ABVS tomogram (L Axilla) view. The homogeneous structure of the breast is clearly visible with duct extension in the subareolar zone. The area of inflammation is a small area on the periphery of the breast (*arrow*)

sinuses and lacunas with inhomogeneous content, and areas of lowered echogenicity without distinct contours (perilobular and periductal infiltration). ABVS in the acute period allows accurate topographical location of the pathological zone for draining the abscess. Abscess formation in the parenchyma is visible as a rounded mass with inhomogeneous liquid contents, distinct capsule, and a peripheral zone of low echogenicity due to infiltration (Fig. 4.53). However, acquisition of ABVS volume data during the acute stage of the disease can be troublesome due to tenderness and pain.

The most common form of non-lactational mastitis in adolescents is suppurative breast cysts. Ultrasound allows us to differentiate the forms of non-lactational mastitis. Focal masses are noted of low echogenicity with clear smooth contours, of round or oval shape, with liquid content surrounded by an area of perifocal inflammation corresponding to the palpable mass, as well as a slight expansion of the lactiferous ducts (Fig. 4.54).

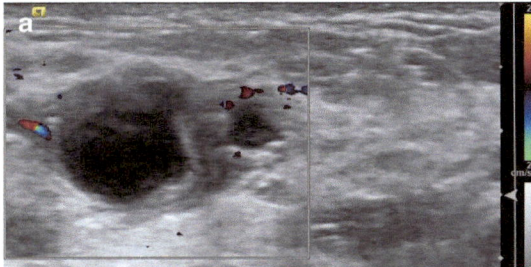
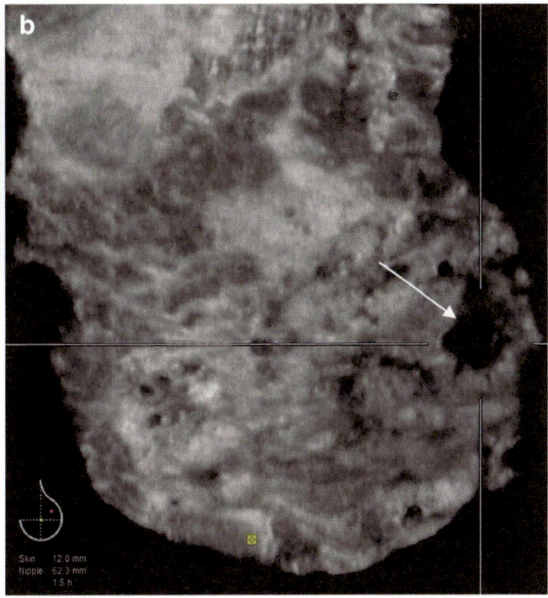

Fig. 4.54 Suppurative breast cyst. Comparison of HHUS and ABVS data. (**a**) HHUS in Color Doppler mode. A small cyst with inhomogeneous internal echoes is seen. The thickened walls are also well detected by HHUS. (**b**) ABVS tomogram in a L Sup view shows striated radiance around the ill-defined nodule in the upper-outer quadrant of the left breast (*white arrow*). The nipple is marked by a *rectangle*

4.7   Breast Implants

The number of women with breast implants is increasing. Augmentation mammoplasty is the most common type of reconstructive surgery worldwide [104]. The first silicone breast prosthesis was developed in 1961 in Texas (USA) [105]. According to the literature, breast implants can be categorized into five implant generations reflecting product development over time. They can all be divided into two major groups: single-lumen silicone implant and double-lumen breast implant. Knowing which implant the patient has can help determine the type of imaging findings to expect in case of rupture. Breast implants may be placed in a subglandular (anterior to the pectoralis major muscle) or subpectoral (posterior to the pectoralis major muscle) location. After placement, a thin fibrous capsule (scar tissue) normally forms around the prosthesis. This occurs around all silicone implants to some degree; however, pronounced fibrous capsule formation causes discomfort and alters the shape of the breast. There are diverse postsurgical complications. These include infection, hematoma, displacement of the implant, fibrosis and capsular contracture, and intra- and extracapsular ruptures. Silicone leakage through the implant shell leads to the development of capsular contracture. According to the literature [106], the most common symptom in breast implant rupture is contour deformity (44 %), followed by displacement (20 %), mass formation (17 %), pain (13 %), and inflammation (3 %).

All breast diseases can also occur in women with implants; among these the most important is breast cancer. The risk of breast cancer is not increased in augmented women [107]; however, implants might interfere with the earliest possible detection of a cancer by altering physical examination of the breast or impairing various imaging techniques [108]. The sensitivity of mammography and US for cancer detection may be reduced in augmented woman [104]. However, the presence of the implant does not seem to decrease the sensitivity of breast MRI [107]. Any palpable abnormalities in patients with implants should be studied with ultrasound or contrast-enhanced MRI. ABVS increased the possibilities of HHUS in evaluation of breast prosthesis.

Physical examination, MRI, mammography, ultrasonography, and exceptionally computed tomography have all been used to diagnose silicone breast implant rupture or other breast abnormalities. Each technique has specific strengths and weaknesses. Physical examination fails to diagnose implant rupture in more than 50% of cases [109].

Mammography is of little value in the assessment of implant integrity, although it may be useful for the assessment of the surrounding breast tissue [104]. In 1988, a special displacement technique for studying breast prosthesis was integrated to facilitate mammography in augmented breasts. Silicone is dense and is not easily penetrated by the X-ray energies used for MMG, which leads to a decrease in image quality, especially in periprosthetic dense band, periprosthetic calcification, and fibrosis. It can be difficult to diagnose intracapsular tears by MMG because of the low sensitivity of the method, reaching 25–30% [104, 110, 111] or 68% according to other authors [112]. But extracapsular rupture and extravasation silicone implant ruptures can be identified. Several studies reported silicone implant rupture during a mammogram due to compression, most probably occurring in women with intracapsular ruptures previous to their mammogram [110–113]. All these factors lower the implementation of MMG in the follow-up process of breast prosthesis.

MRI is the most accurate technique in the evaluation of implant integrity. Its sensitivity for rupture is between 80 and 90%, and its specificity is between 90 and 97% [110, 112–114]. MRI's usefulness derives from its ability to suppress or emphasize the signal from water, fat, or especially silicone. Its high spatial and soft-tissue resolutions make it ideal for the characterization of breast implants [114].

US is the method of choice for the follow-up of patients after mammoplasty. US does not use ionizing radiation, is noninvasive and safe, and can be repeated for follow-up studies [115]. A completely negative US examination for implant rupture limits the application of MMG and MRI to cases suspicious on US [106, 114]. However, the method has several limitations that reduce its sensitivity. One of the major weaknesses is that US is operator dependent; the second, reverberation artifacts in the anterior aspect of the implant could be confused with abnormalities; and the third, attenuation of the US beam by silicone hinders the evaluation of the back wall of an implant and the tissue posterior to it [112]. With conventional HHUS, it is difficult to measure the diameter of the implant exactly due to the short transducer field of view. Additional use of panoramic view causes distortions in the measurements due to the concave surface of the implant and does not provide global information of prosthesis structure and location that can be obtained with a three-dimensional reconstruction on ABVS [105].

ABVS technology allows representation of global breast anatomy with the prosthesis in one scan, including precise information of its posterior contour and the surrounding tissues. Multiplanar reconstruction mode helps in measurement of distances from the anterior to the posterior implant surface and accurately determines the smoothness of its contours, the presence and depth of radial folds, the status of the implant's shell and of the fibrous capsule, and the presence of silicone granulomas. One can easily see the internal surface of the implant, especially the posterior wall using 3D coronal slices because silicone is anechoic and give excellent possibilities to look through it.

4.7.1   Normal Breast Implant

An intact implant has an uninterrupted shell and fibrous capsule adjacent to the breast parenchyma. Sonographically it is characterized by anechoic lumen and clearly traceable smooth contours. The fibrous capsule is formed around the implant in about 1 month after mammoplasty and is visualized as a thin hyperechoic line. Radial folds present as echogenic lines that extend from the periphery to the interior of the implant. These folds and periprosthetic fluid are considered normal variants of breast implants.

With ABVS coronal slices, the implant's internal surface can be clearly studied. Bilateral side-by-side comparative ABVS tomograms help in evaluation of prosthesis symmetry. Coronal slices close to the nipple area show anteriorly located breast tissue in a similar way as without implants. And the deeper slices give comparison of the prosthesis. On the deeper frontal slices, we can also measure the thickness, diameter, and maximum length of the implant. The shape of the implant is clearly visible, as spherical, oval, or droplike with ABVS. The total view of the posterior surface at ABVS tomogram is comparable to that in the surface mode.

4.7.2 Capsular Contracture

As part of the physiologic response to a foreign material (implant), the body also reacts by forming a fibrous capsule around the material (i.e., the breast implant). Capsular contraction following implantation of breast prostheses occurs in 2–33 % of patients undergoing breast augmentation [115]. This complication can develop weeks or years after implantation of breast prosthesis; however, approximately 60 % of capsular contracture occurs within 6 months and 90 % within 12 months postoperatively [116]. This complication is a huge problem for breast cancer patients undergoing reconstructive surgery.

Capsular contracture is characterized by fibrosis and contraction of the breast capsule which can affect woman with breast implants. Capsular contracture is the second-most common complication after hematoma and infection. It is caused by excessive scar tissue around the implant that tightens and squeezes the implant so that infoldings of the shell begin. Pronounced fibrous capsule formation causes discomfort and alters the shape of the breast, reduces it in volume, and causes asymmetry and contour irregularity, usually detected by the patient during self-examination.

When the normal US reveal no changes of the breast implant and clearly visualize only its front surface, the ABVS tomogram shows expressed radial folds and subfolds on the posterior surface of the implant, which indicates the formation of capsular contracture, a complication of mammoplasty (Fig. 4.55). Latero-medial slices show the posterior contour of the implant, undulation, or folds more clearly. Multiplanar reconstruction allows more accurate measurement of the depth of radial folds and easily identifies radial folds of the implant (Fig. 4.56).

The severity of capsular contracture is classified by Baker's classification. It is based on visual evaluation of the implant and on palpation data. There are four grades of breast capsular contracture—Baker grades I–IV. For this system, a soft but visible implant (grade I) and an implant with mild firmness (grade II) are considered good or excellent outcomes. Initial signs of contracture (Baker classes I–II) correspond to fibrous capsule thickening more than 0.3–0.5 mm, with a depth of the radial folds not more than 0.2–0.6 cm [105]. An implant with moderate firmness (grade III) may require treatment if symptomatic and class IV classification, with an excessively firm and symptomatic breast result in a significantly poor aesthetic result [117]. Significant capsular contracture (Baker class III–IV) is characterized by the spherical shape of the silicone implant, more than 0.9 mm thickening of the capsule, the rough contour deformation due to the deep radial folds sized more than 0.6–0.8 cm, the presence of stable capsule infoldings, enhanced echogenicity, and blurred contour. These changes are clearly visible during multiplanar reconstruction analysis of latero-medial views of the breasts on an ABVS tomogram (Fig. 4.57).

The changing of the implant shape may be the only sign of capsular contracture (Fig. 4.58). Class III–IV capsular contracture is clinically significant as its detection is an indication for implant replacement. In areas of permanent contracture of the silicone implant, the shell is thinned and calcified with the loss of elasticity and strain formation. When the inner implant shell strains, the content of the prosthesis becomes nonuniform, and if the shape and thickness of the implant are not changed, it is very difficult to determine the location of the strain. The shell becomes discontinuous and blurred. Strains are considered a precursor of tears [105].

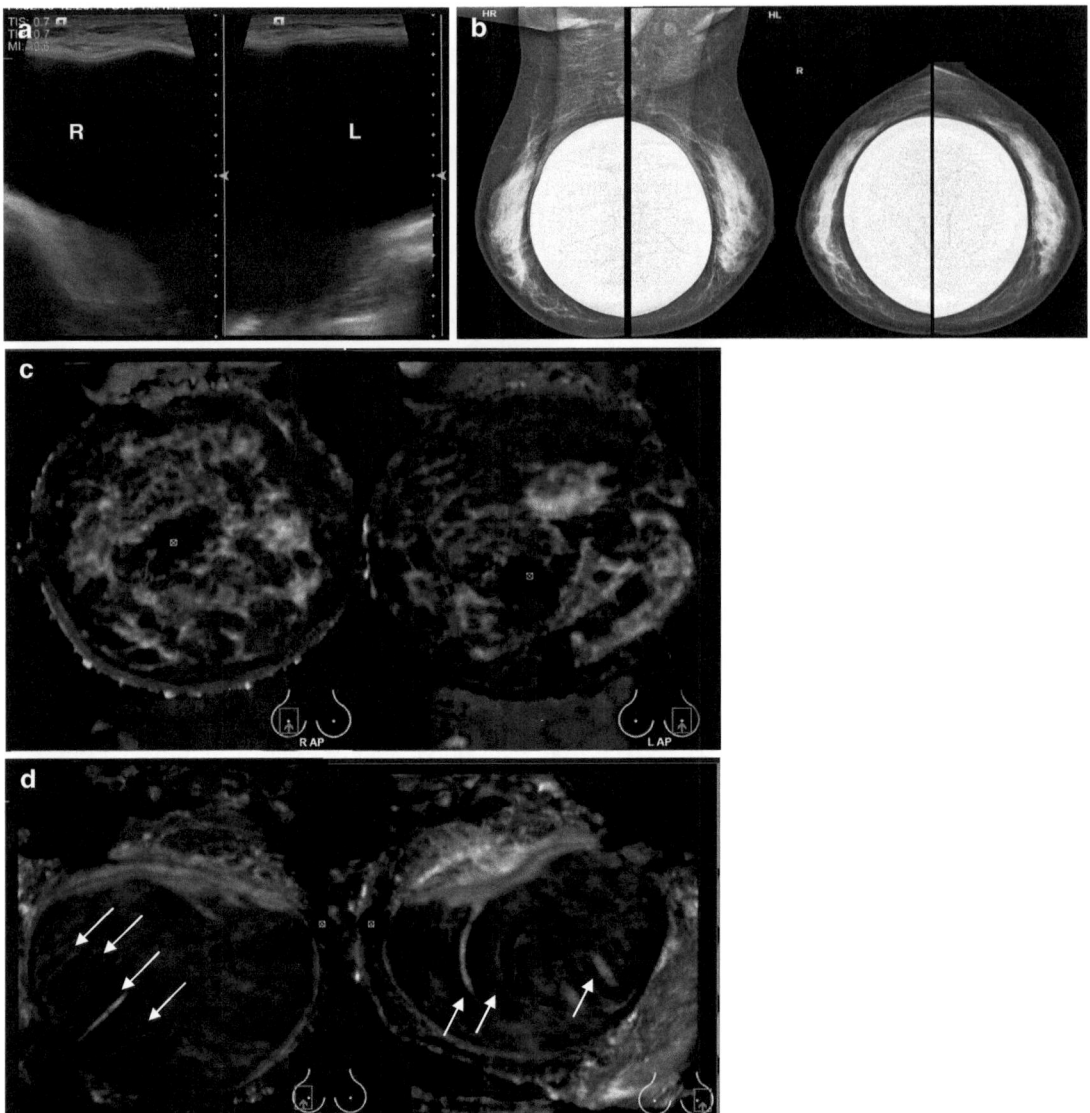

Fig. 4.55 Five-year history of bilateral augmentation mammoplasty for cosmetic reasons with silicone implants. Early stage of capsular contracture (I–II). Moderate folding of the implants smoothed after slight pressure. Comparison of HHUS, MMG, and ABVS performance. (**a**) Bilateral HHUS. Right (*R*) and left (*L*) breast silicone implants. Undulation of the contours. The absence of capsular contracture. (**b**) X-ray mammogram. Bilateral side-by-side comparison of the breasts. Subpectoral placed implants are visible. The preserved glandular tissue is displaced anteriorly from the implants. No signs of capsular contracture. (**c**) Bilateral ABVS coronal views (R AP and L AP) on the level of glandular tissue. Moderate asymmetry of the glandular tissue development is noted. (**d**) Bilateral ABVS tomograms in oblique latero-medial views (R Lat and L Lat) provide an endoscopic view of the implant's internal surface. The posterior surface of both implants has linear folds (*arrows*) and demonstrate a "rat-tail sign" not visible on usual 2D scan and X-ray mammogram suggesting early capsular contracture. The nipples are marked by a *rectangle*

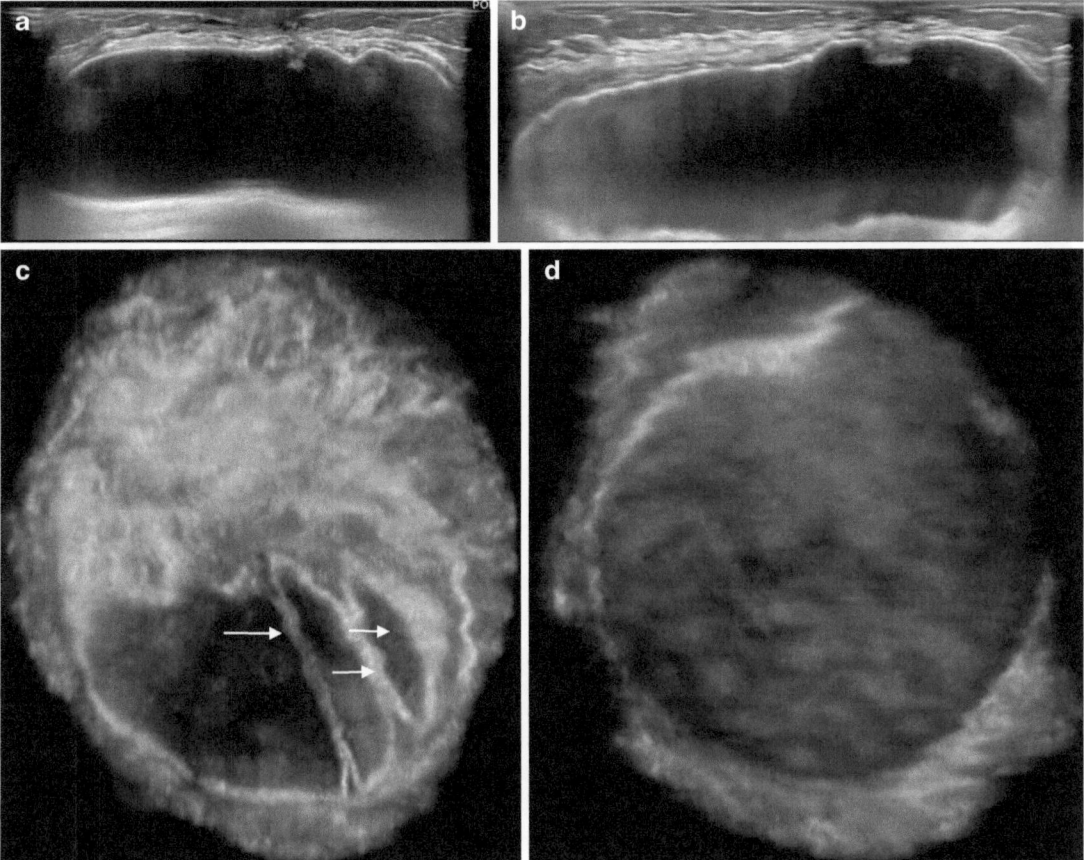

Fig. 4.56 Four-year post-bilateral breast augmentation. Capsular contracture formation. Comparison of HHUS and ABVS images. (**a**, **b**) HHUS. Right breast implant (**a**). Left breast implant (**b**). Waving of the contours without clear evidence of capsular contracture. The roughness of the anterior surface of the implants is noted. Echogenicity of the left implant is increased. (**c**, **d**) ABVS images in the coronal projection. Right implant (**c**), left implant (**d**). ABVS clearly shows signs of capsular contracture in the right breast prosthesis. Marked asymmetry of the implant's shape. Significant infolding of the posterior and lateral surfaces (*arrows*) of the right implant, "rat-tail sign." Round shape and smooth posterior surface of the left implant

4.7.3   Intracapsular Implant Rupture

Intracapsular implant rupture is defined as rupture of the implant shell with silicone leakage that does not macroscopically extend beyond the fibrous capsule. The dense fibrous capsule holds the gel inside and prevents the expressed change of breast shape.

Intracapsular rupture cannot be identified by mammography.

MRI findings could be divided into definitive signs of rupture and possible signs of rupture. All of them can be easily transferred to ABVS modality as well. Contour deformity with bulging (so-called rat-tail sign), irregular margin, blurring of the borders, mixed inflating echoes inside the implant, "noose sign" or "keyhole sign" or "teardrop sign," and small invaginations where the two membranes do not touch are possible signs of rupture. Definitive signs of breast implant rupture are subcapsular lines, running almost parallel to the fibrous capsule and just beneath it, "linguine sign" on MRI and "step-ladder sign" on US, folded wavy multidirectional lines within the silicone gel, and "railroad track sign," two parallel lines in close proximity form-

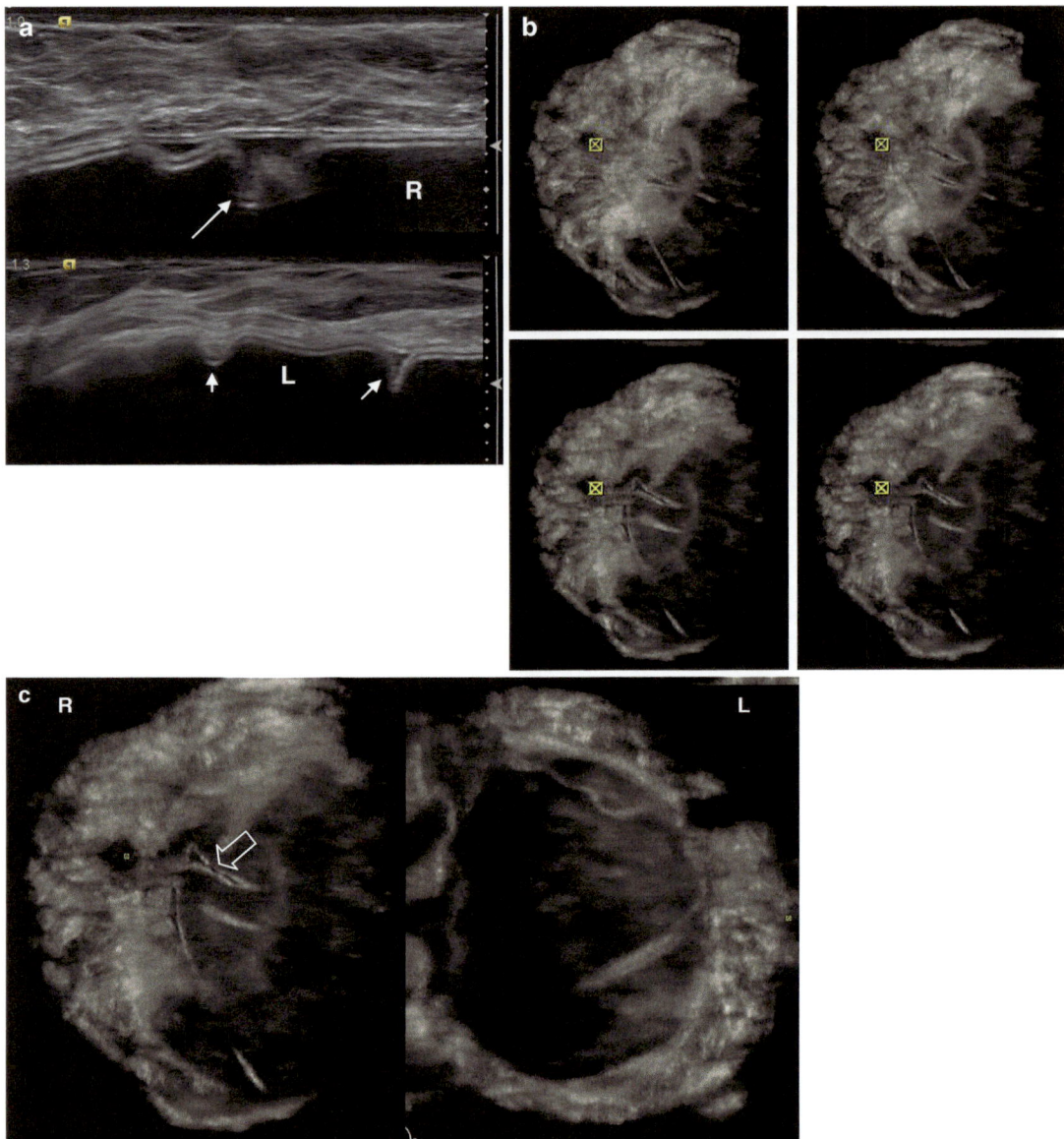

Fig. 4.57 Ten-year post-bilateral breast augmentation. Double-lumen breast implants. Capsular contraction. Comparison of HHUS and ABVS images. (**a**) HHUS. Right silicone implant (*R*), upper part; left silicone implant (*L*), lower part. Folding of the anterior shell (*arrows*) in both implants, radial folds. (**b**) ABVS in multislice reconstruction mode of the right breast. Implant with excessive radial folds. The nipple is marked by a *rectangle*. (**c**) Bilateral ABVS in latero-medial oblique views. Image analysis on the workstation. (*R* right implant, *L* left implant). Significant folding of the anterior, posterior, and lateral surfaces of both implants, "keyhole sign" (*open arrow*). Fibrous capsule without any signs of thickening and increased echogenicity

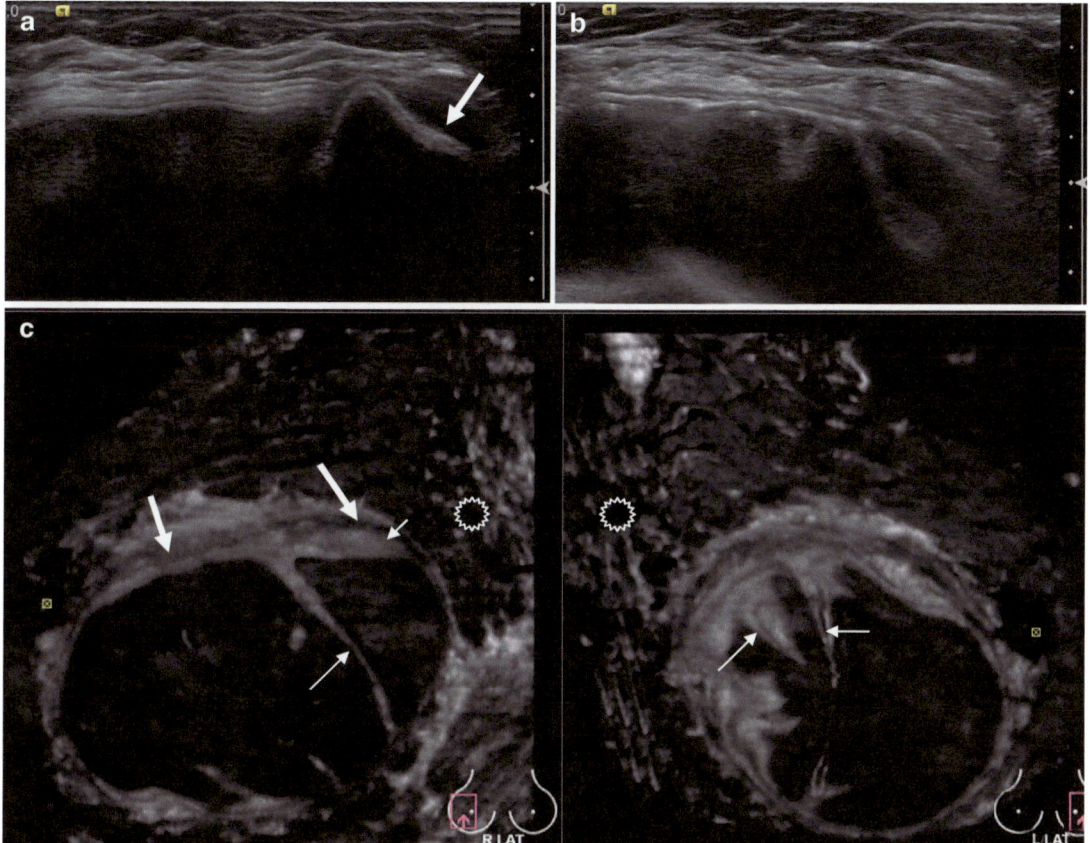

Fig. 4.58 A woman with bilateral silicone breast implants, 8-year postimplantation. Submammary implants. Severe capsular contraction. Comparison of HHUS and ABVS data. (**a, b**) HHUS. Right implant (**a**), left implant (**b**). Significant radial folds with formation of "infolding" and a serous liquid between the implant and the fibrous capsule (*thick arrows*). (**c**) Bilateral ABVS tomogram in latero-medial oblique view (*R LAT* right breast implant, *L LAT* left breast implant). Asymmetry of implant shapes with shrinkage of the left implant. "Keyhole sign" and "teardrop sign" forms (*thin arrows*). Thickening of fibrous capsule depicted as zones of increased echogenicity (*thick arrows*). ABVS clearly shows the pectoralis muscle layers behind the implants (*asterisk*)

ing a double-contoured subcapsular line within the silicone gel outside the implant shell. An ABVS tomogram also helps in assessing the shape and the contours of the implant (Fig. 4.59).

4.7.4   Extracapsular Implant Rupture

Extracapsular rupture damages the fibrous capsule, which in earlier implant generations allowed silicone to leak through the site of damage into the surrounding breast tissue, forming silicone granulomas. Modern implants use high-viscosity gel that cannot move beyond the implant. However, it causes a visual change of the breast form and allows easy clinical identification of the implant tear. A leak of the gel outside the fibrous capsule is a violation of the integrity of the prosthesis.

Because MMG can easily detect free silicone within the breast parenchyma, an extracapsular silicone implant rupture can be identified. Specific mammographic evidence of implant rupture is extravasation of silicone outside the implant shell [115].

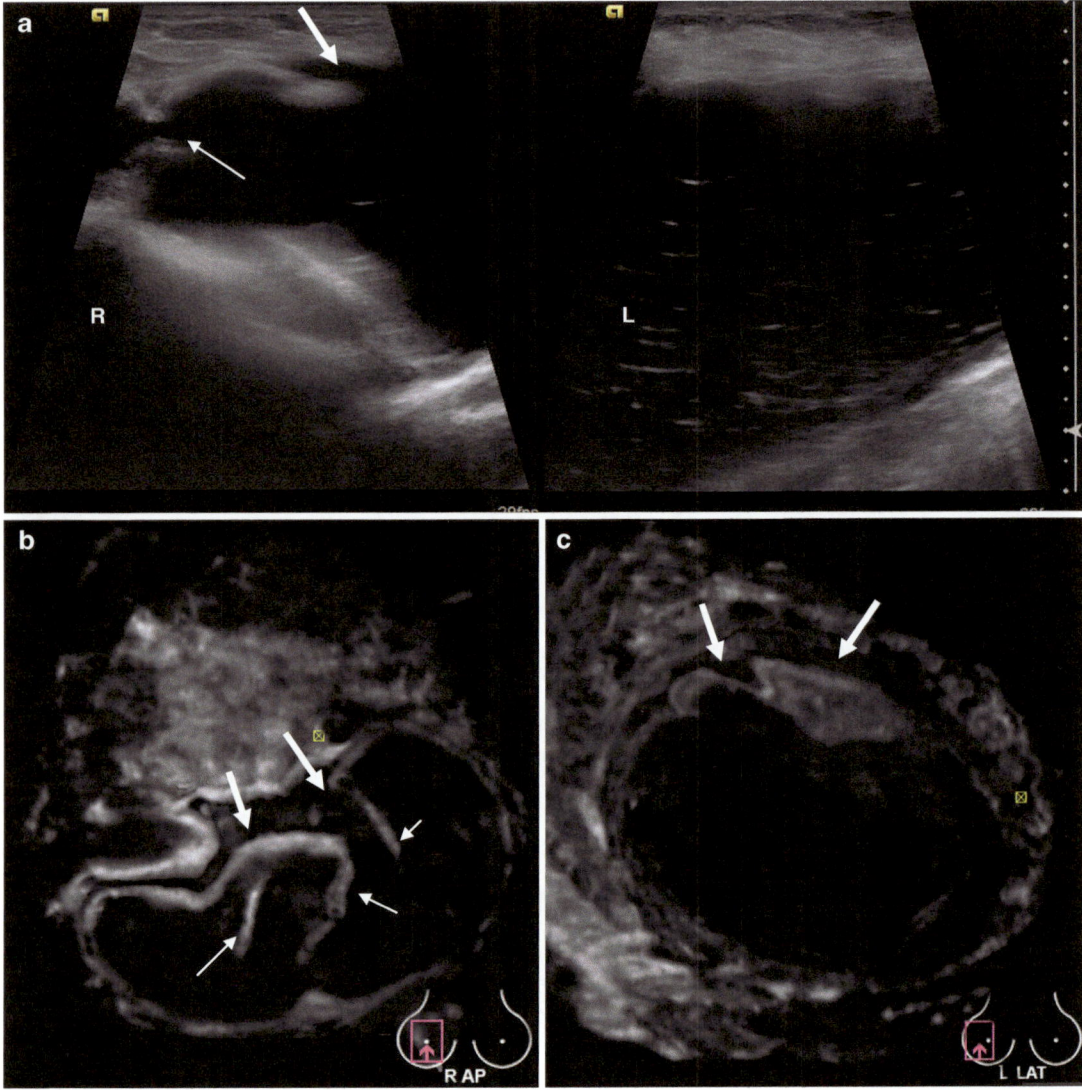

Fig. 4.59 Intracapsular rupture of breast implants, confirmed at surgery. 12-year post-bilateral breast augmentation. Comparison of HHUS and ABVS. (**a**) Bilateral HHUS. Right silicone implant (*R*), left part; left silicone implant (*L*), right part. Collapsed right silicone implant. Changes in internal structure of the left implant. Significant folding with "stepladder sign" in the right side (*thin arrows*) and periimplant aggregations of the gel (*thick arrows*). (**b, c**) ABVS tomograms. Right breast

implant (**b**), left breast implant (**c**). *R AP* anteroposterior coronal view of the right breast implant, latero-medial oblique view of the left breast (*R AP* right breast, *L LAT* left breast). Asymmetry of implant shapes with collapse of the right implant. Thickening of the fibrous capsule. "Stepladder sign" (*thick arrows*) or "linguine sign" (*thin arrows*). Complex folds of the left implant, silicone leakage confirmed surgically in the left prosthesis

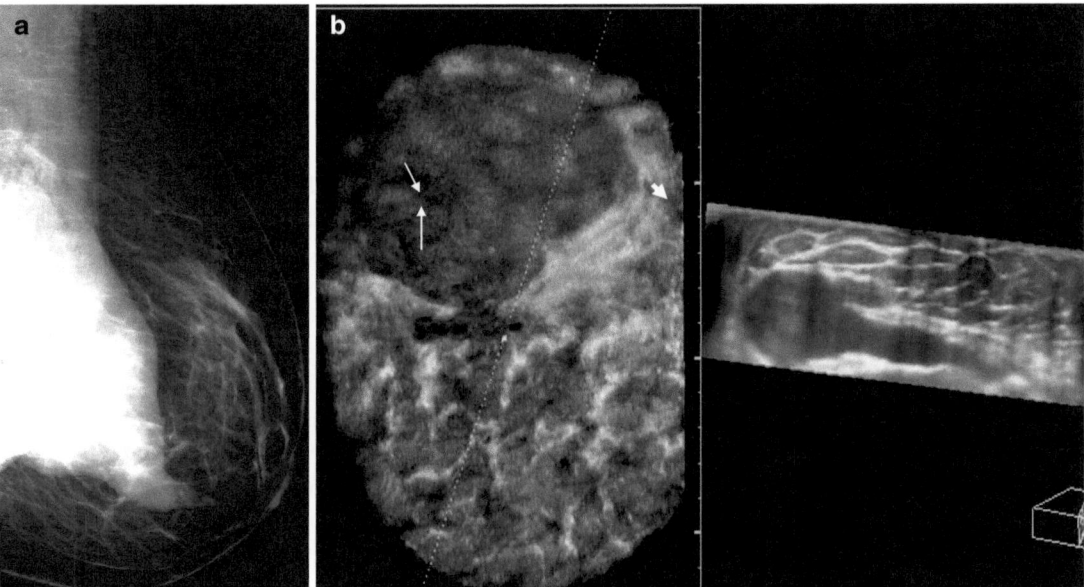

Fig. 4.60 Extracapsular rupture of the left implant in woman with a history of breast cancer and radiotherapy. Comparison of MMG and ABVS data. (**a**) X-ray mammogram. Implant shape defect with extravasation of silicone in the breast tissue and silicon granuloma formation. (**b**) ABVS. Biplanar comparison mode. A defect in the fibrous capsule (*thin arrows*) is clearly seen on the coronal (L AP) and sagittal (L Ax) views. The image is sliced through the ruptured capsule. Coronal slice shows the large leak of silicone in the breast tissue (*thick arrow*) with the formation of siliconoma

A specific US sign of extracapsular rupture is a so-called "snowstorm" picture which emphasizes the free silicone in the breast tissue. The presence of silicone granulomas gives an increase in echogenicity of the entire breast parenchyma.

An ABVS tomogram shows a total violation of the contours of the implant and its tapering. Multiplanar reconstruction helps in identification of the silicone leakage (Fig. 4.60). Sometimes the leaked silicone causes changes in acoustic properties of the breast tissue and makes it difficult to visualize the breast in the usual B-mode. In such cases MRI is suggested.

4.8   Postoperative Breast

Breast surgery today ranges from mamma reduction to augmentation and from mastopexia to mammoplasty with the restoration of breasts lost to disease or trauma [119]. Improvement of X-ray diagnosis, surgical techniques, and adjuvant therapy of cancer has led to an increase in organ preserving surgery in oncomammology. Multivariate analysis showed that local recurrence in the scar occurs most often in young women up to 45-years-old with infiltrative ductal carcinoma localized in the central or at the margin of the upper quadrants. Observation in this group of patients should be carried out with the utmost care. The recurrence rate in the preserved breast varies from 2 to 10 % within 5 years and from 5 to 15 % over 10 years [120–122]. Even in the absence of metastases in regional lymph nodes, the relapse rate reaches 25–30 % [121]. Therefore, the remaining breast tissue requires careful observation throughout the subsequent life of the patient.

Identification of recurrent breast cancer can be difficult against the background of postoperative and post-radiation scar deformation [123]. Scarring and fibrosis often complicate the early detection of breast cancer recurrence in the area of primary surgery and its differential diagnosis with a variety of postoperative and/ or post-radiation local changes [119]. We must know these postoperative conditions and the characteristics of the postoperative complications to distinguish recurrence from benign conditions.

An excision site may exhibit defects, cyst formation, or scar-like images. Fat necrosis is one of the benign postoperative disorders. It is noninfectious fat degeneration by inflammatory changes or phenomena such as postsurgical disturbance of blood flow. Evaluation of the presence or absence of residual disease may often be difficult. After radiation therapy, skin thickening and skin edema may be seen. Conventional ultrasound does not always display the deeper areas of the gland clearly, due to the pronounced attenuation of the echo signal. Dystrophic calcification occurs in degenerated or necrotic tissue. The diagnosis of benignity is not so difficult with its characteristic coarse calcification. But, during the forming progress of coarse calcification, amorphous calcification or pleomorphic calcification may be seen, and definitive diagnosis by X-ray mammography is difficult; thus, appropriate follow-up by US or MRI is recommended for these cases.

Microcalcifications in the postoperative scar area may be one of the first signs of breast cancer recurrence. In some cases, it can manifest itself as a spiculated lesion, simulating a picture of breast cancer recurrence. Approximately 30 % of

cases of breast cancer recurrence according to X-ray mammography are shown to be benign by intraoperative biopsy [123]. Spiculated lesions can be the result of benign or malignant processes as well. These include sclerosing adenosis, postsurgical scar, radial scar, post-traumatic oil cysts, and infiltrating ductal carcinoma [124]. The radial scar is a stellate lesion, which mammographically can be indistinguishable from a carcinoma. It also has a radiolucent central core, elongated radiating spicules, and infrequent calcification. Sonographically radial scars are not diagnostic either. The lesions produce ill-defined margins with poor echogenicity and shadowing. MRI did not differentiate benign radial scars from those harboring malignancy [125]. ABVS will also show the stellate pattern if it is presented mammographically, but without specific differentiation from IDC. Recommendations are to excise all stellate lesions if they are seen in all three projections on ABVS as cancer cannot be excluded.

Cancer can also be erroneously diagnosed in patients with a postoperative scar after sectoral resection of fibroadenoma or after surgery for mastitis, also visible as streaking in the scar area similar to that in malignancy [119]. Ultrasound is complementary to mammography for the diagnosis of local recurrence of breast cancer. A postoperative scar is hypoechoic on conventional B-mode ultrasound with distal acoustic shadowing, similar to a tumor nodule. Power Doppler helps to evaluate the presence of blood flow in the tumors. But if it is a small tumor, Doppler can be insensitive in flow detection [125]. Elastography sometimes cannot differentiate fibrosis from a tumor also because both zones are mapped as a stiffer area. A potential solution for this is the use of ABVS with volume multiplanar scanning. Unlike breast cancer, the postoperative scar shows "retraction" phenomenon only in one view on an ABVS tomogram and on others (sagittal, axial) shows only a hypoechoic scar line from the nipple area deep into the glandular tissue (Fig. 4.61). This feature can be used for differential diagnosis of the two generically

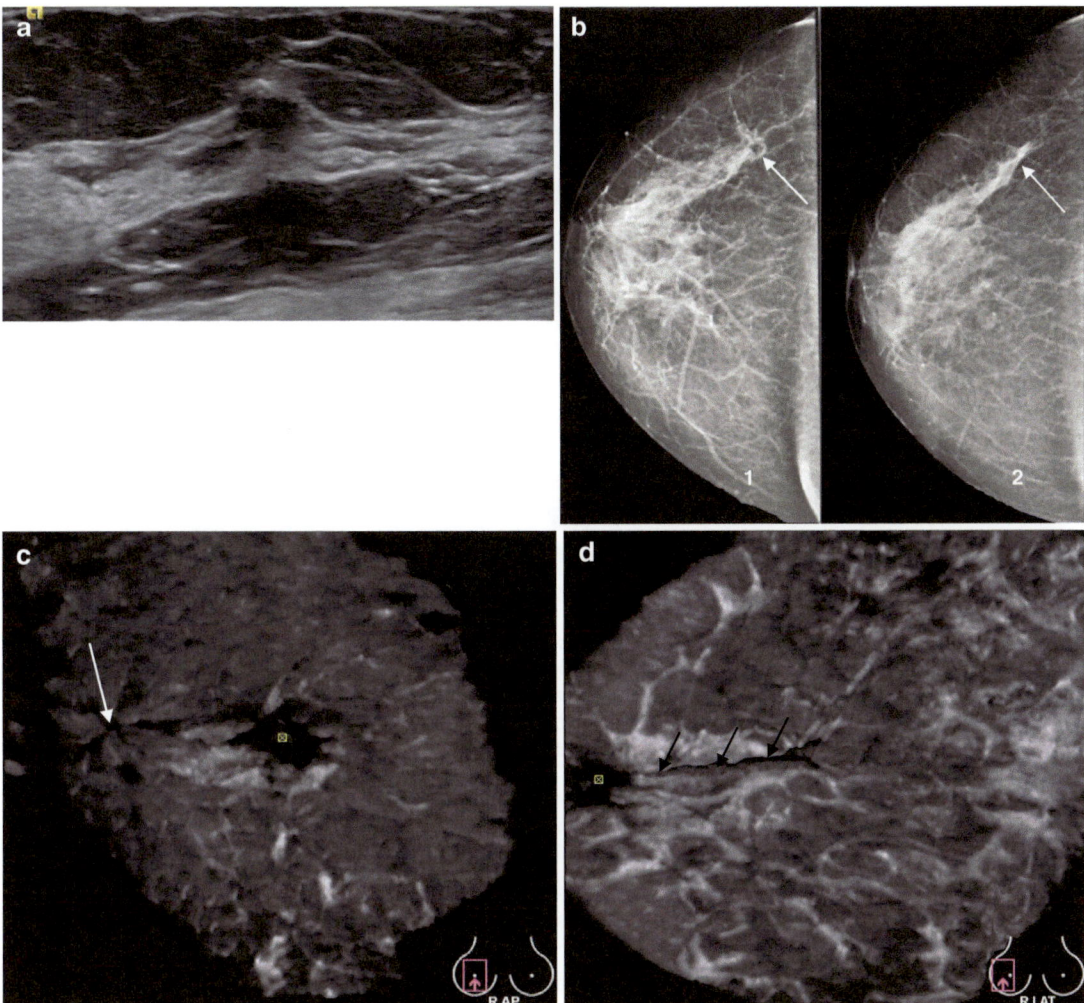

Fig. 4.61 Postoperative scar after mastitis in the right breast in a 68-year-old female. Comparison of HHUS, ABVS, and mammographic appearance. (**a**) A hypoechoic area with indistinct contours and moderate distal shadowing is seen on HHUS. (**b**) Comparative mammograms in direct craniocaudal projection. Left part (1) at the time of the study, right part (2) 1 year after the study. Radiolucent nodule with stellate appearance and a radiating pattern on the border of the outer quadrants (*arrow*) is clearly seen. One year after the study—reduction of the size of the stellate radiolucent area (*arrow*) in a year (2) is characteristic of scarring. (**c**, **d**) ABVS tomograms in two different projections: Coronal anteroposterior view (**c**), latero-medial oblique (**d**). A spiculated lesion with evidently prominent radiate lines in the border of the outer quadrants of the right breast (*white arrow*). On the perpendicular plane in latero-medial oblique position, this area corresponds to the hypoechoic line and derives from the nipple to the deep parts of the gland (*black arrows*). No lesions with radiate pattern are seen

different processes: postoperative fibrosis and cancer recurrence in the scar.

Sectoral resection causes a significant change in the breast parenchyma. If the glandular tissue still exists in the rest of the breast, fatty tissue will appear in the resected area. By comparing the changes with the contralateral gland, one can reveal the structural deformity of the glandular pattern in the postoperational breast, regardless of the period after the surgery (Fig. 4.62).

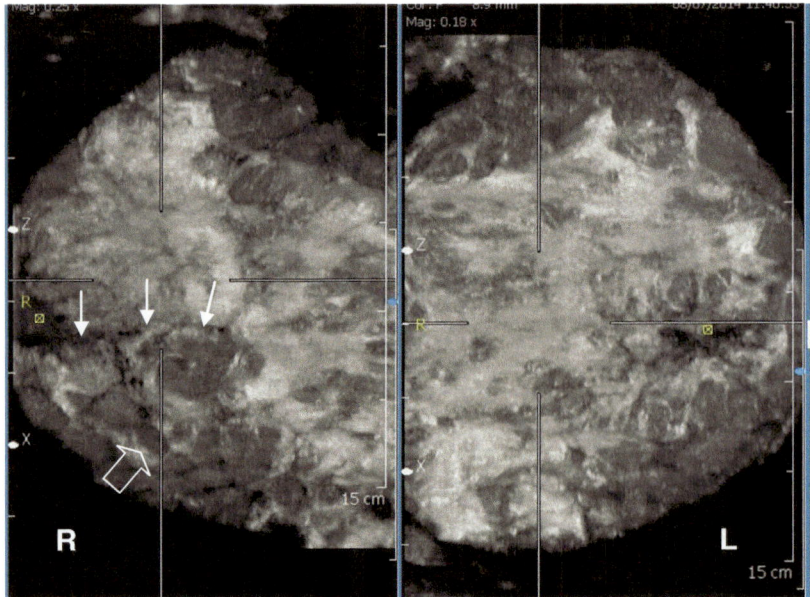

Fig. 4.62 Postoperative right breast. History of a sectoral resection 5 years prior to the examination in a 39-year-old woman. ABVS image analysis on a workstation. Bilateral comparison of the latero-medial oblique views of the right (*R*) and left (*L*) breasts. Asymmetry of the glandular pattern is seen. The absence of the glandular component in the lower areas in the right breast (*open arrow*), and a shrunk area is clearly seen with a substitution by fatty tissue (*arrows*)

Scarring in the glandular tissue can be present as a stellate pattern or tissue retraction especially after excision of large masses or lumpectomy. The scar deformity and degenerative processes can form cysts around the surgical area. Comparison of mammography and ABVS tomogram images helps to understand the nature of these changes more accurately (Fig. 4.63).

Reduction mammoplasty results in a small volume and displacement of the preserved glandular tissue, with asymmetry of the breast structure and with frequent formation of linear strands, oil cysts, and calcification. An ABVS tomogram significantly helps in the evaluation of the glandular structure after surgery (Fig. 4.64).

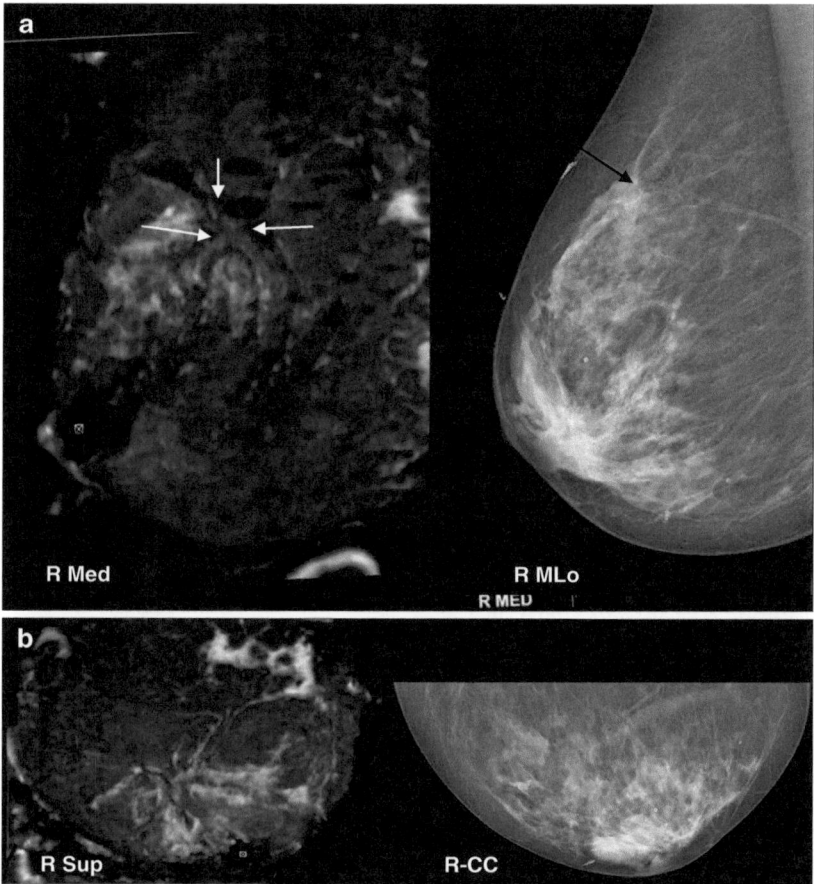

Fig. 4.63 Postoperative breast scar deformity of the right breast after large fibroadenoma excision. ABVS and mammographic comparison of the corresponding projections. Computer data processing for matching oblique mediolateral views (**a, b**)—direct craniocaudal views. (**a**) Comparison of ABVS (*left part*) and X-ray mammography (*right part*). An area with severe radiance is found in the upper-outer quadrant of the right breast (*white arrows*). Note tissue retraction and cystic formation around the scarred deformed tissue. The X-ray mammogram also shows the scar area, marked with a black arrow. (**b**) Comparison of ABVS (*left part*) and X-ray mammography (*right part*). The same pattern of the lesion as described above is seen in the outer portion of the breast

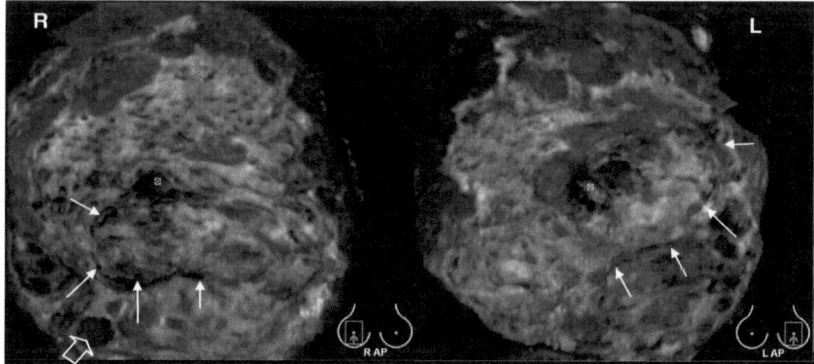

Fig. 4.64 Breast glandular tissue deformity after bilateral reduction mammoplasty in a 38-year-old patient. ABVS performance on the workstation. Comparison of the coronal anteroposterior views of the right (*R*) and left (*L*) breasts. The scar line is clearly visible (*arrows*) in both breasts. Fibroadenoma was found in the right breast (*open arrow*) with a typical hyperechoic rim

Literature

1. Chinyama CN (2014) The normal female breast in benign breast diseases. Springer, Berlin/Heidelberg, pp 1–7
2. Burdina LM (1993) Clinical and X-ray features of breast disease in gynecological patients of reproductive age with neuroendocrine pathology. Abstract of Dr. Med. Sci. Thesis. Moscow (book in Russian)
3. Serov VN, Taghiyev TT, Prilepskaya VN (1999) Diagnostics of breast pathology. Gynecology 1:6–10 (article in Russian)
4. Moore KL, Dalley AF, Agur AMR (2006) Clinically oriented anatomy, 5th edn. Lippincott Williams & Wilkins, Philadelphia
5. Widmaier EP, Raff H, Strang KT (2006) Vander's human physiology: the mechanisms of body function, 10th edn. McGraw-Hill, Boston
6. Mansel RE, Webster DJT, Sweetland HM (eds) (2009) Breast anatomy and physiology. In: Hughes, Mansel & Webster's benign disorders and disease of the breast, 3rdedn. Saunders Elsevier, China, pp 25–40
7. Zabolotskaya NV, Zabolotskii VS (1997) Ultrasound mammography. Academic atlas. Strom, Moscow (book in Russian)
8. Kharchenko VP, Rozhkova NI (2000) X-ray diagnosis of breast diseases, treatment, and rehabilitation. Issue 1. Strom, Moscow, p 56 (book in Russian)
9. Boyd NF, Guo H, Martin LJ et al (2007) Mammographic density and the risk and detection of breast cancer. N Engl J Med 356:227–236
10. Rozhkova NI (2014) X-ray diagnosis in mammology: guide for physicians. SpecIzdat, Moscow, p 36 (book in Russian)
11. Foster ME, Garrahan N, Williams S (1988) Fibroadenoma of the breast: a clinical and pathological study. J R Coll Surg Edinb 33:16–19
12. Hunter TB, Roberts CC, Hunt KR et al (1996) Occurrence of fibroadenomas in post-menopausal women referred for breast biopsy. J Am Geriatr Soc 44:61–64
13. Dent DM, Cant PJ (1989) Fibroadenoma. World J Surg 13:706–710
14. Matz D, Kerivan L, Reintgen M et al (2013) Breast preservation in women with giant juvenile fibroadenomas. Clin Breast Cancer 13:219–222
15. Zonderland HM (2002) Sonography of the breast. In: Dronkers DJ, Hendricks JHCL, Holland R, Rosenbusch G (eds) The practice of mammography. Thieme, Stuttgart, pp 151–169
16. Tabar L, Dean PB (1985) Circumscribed lesion. In: Teaching atlas of mammography, 2nd edn. Thieme, Stuttgart, pp 18–56
17. Sickles EA (1994) Nonpalpable, circumscribed, noncalcified solid breast masses: likelihood of malignancy based on lesion size and age of patient. Radiology 192:439–442
18. Yamaguchi R, Tanaka M, Mizushima YMT et al (2011) Myxomatous fibroadenoma of the breast: correlation with clinic-pathologic and radiologic features. Hum Pathol 42:419–423
19. Heywang-Koebrunner SH, Dershaw DD, Schreer I (2001) Benign tumors. In: Diagnostic breast imaging. Thieme, Stuttgart, pp 209–235
20. Chen L, Chen Y (2013) Comparative study of automated breast 3-D ultrasound and handheld B-mode ultrasound for differentiation of benign and malignant breast masses. Ultrasound Med Biol 39(10):1735–1742
21. Bernstein L, Deapen D, Ross RK (1993) The descriptive epidemiology of malignant cystosarcoma phyllodes tumors of the breast. Cancer 71:3020–3024
22. Abe M, Miyata S, Nishimura S et al (2011) Malignant transformation of breast fibroadenoma to malignant phyllodes tumor: long-term outcome of 36 malignant phyllodes tumors. Breast Cancer 18:268–272
23. Wojcinski S, Farrokh A, Hille U et al (2011) The automated breast volume scanner (ABVS): initial experiences in lesion detection compared with conventional handheld B-mode ultrasound: pilot study of 50 cases. Int J Womens Health 13:337–346
24. Gazhonova V, Yefremova M, Potkin S (2015) Breast cancer evaluation in women with dense breast with 3D Automated Breast Volume Sonography. In EPOS electronic presentation on-line system ECR 2015/doi:C-028010.1594/ecr2015/C-0280. doi-link:http://dx.doi.org/10.1594/ecr2015/C-0280
25. Wellings SR, Alpers CE (1987) Apocrine cystic metaplasia: subgross pathology and prevalence in cancer-associated versus random autopsy breasts. Hum Pathol 18:381–386
26. Drukker BN, deMendonca WC (1987) Fibrocystic change and fibrocystic disease of the breast. Obstet Gynecol Clin North Am 14:685–702
27. Warner JK, Kumar D, Berg WA (1998) Apocrine metaplasia: mammographic and sonographic appearances. Am J Roentgenol 170:1375–1379
28. Agnantis NJ, Mahera H, Maounis N et al (1992) Immunohistochemical study of ras and myconcoproteins in apocrine breast lesions with and without papillomatosis. Eur J Gynecol Oncol 13:309–315
29. Tabar L, Dean PB (1985) Circumscribed lesion; calcifications. In: Teaching atlas of mammography. Georg Thieme Verlag, Stuttgart/New York, p 18, pp 172–210
30. Trofimova TN, Solntseva IA (2000) Possibilities of ultrasonography in the diagnosis of diffuse fibrocystic mastopathy. Sonoace Int 6:79–85 (article in Russian)
31. Heywang-Koebrunner SH, Dershaw DD, Schreer I (2001) Cysts; inflammatory conditions. In: Diagnostic breast imaging. Thieme, Stuttgart/New York, pp 197–208; 236–251
32. Lanyi M (2003) Lesions of the internal ducts and lobules. In: Mammography, diagnosis and pathological analysis. Springer, Berlin/Heidelberg/New York, pp 28–79

33. Okello J, Kisembo H, Bugeza S et al (2014) Breast cancer detection using sonography in women with mammographically dense breast. BMC Med Imaging 14:41. doi:10.1186/s12880-014-0041-0
34. Tabar L, Vitak B, Chen TH et al (2011) Swedish two-county trial: impact of mammographic screening on breast cancer mortality during 3 decades. Radiology 260:658–663
35. Kuhl CK, Schrading S, Leutner CC et al (2005) Mammography, breast ultrasound, and magnetic resonance imaging for surveillance of women at high familial risk for breast cancer. J Clin Oncol 23:8469–8476
36. Berg WA, Blume JD, Cormack JB et al (2008) Combined screening with ultrasound and mammography vs mammography alone in women at elevated risk of breast cancer. JAMA 299:2151–2163
37. Zonderland HM, Coerkamp EG, Hermans J et al (1999) Diagnosis of breast cancer: contribution of US as an adjunct to mammography. Radiology 213:413–422
38. Kelly KM, Dean J, Comulada WS et al (2010) Breast cancer detection using automated whole breast ultrasound and mammography in radiographically dense breasts. Eur Radiol 20:734–742
39. Kelly KM, Dean J, Lee SJ et al (2010) Breast cancer detection: radiologists' performance using mammography with and without automated whole-breast ultrasound. Eur Radiol 20:2557–2564
40. Shin HJ, Kim HH, Cha JH et al (2011) Automated ultrasound of the breast for diagnosis: interobserver agreement on lesion detection and characterization. AJR Am J Roentgenol 197:747–754
41. Chen L, Chen Y, Diao XN et al (2013) Comparative study of automated breast 3-D ultrasound and hand-held B-mode ultrasound for differentiation of benign and malignant breast masses. Ultrasound Med Bio l39(10):1735–1742
42. Tozaki M, Fukuma E (2010) Accuracy of determining preoperative cancer extent measured by automated breast ultrasonography. Jpn J Radiol 13(10):771–773
43. Chae EY, Shin HJ, Kim HJ et al (2013) Diagnostic performance of automated breast ultrasound as a replacement for a hand-held second-look ultrasound for breast lesions detected initially on magnetic resonance imaging. Ultrasound Med Biol 39:2246–2254
44. Jacobs OE, Rozhkova NI, Maso ML et al (2014) The experience of breast virtual sonography. Ann Roentgenol Radiol 1:23–32 (article in Russian)
45. Gazhonova VE, Bachurina EM, Khlustina EM et al (2014) Automatic sonotomography of mammary glands (3D ABVS). Part 1. Integration of ABVS method in the radiological imaging standards. Polyclinic. Radiology 42–48 (article in Russian)
46. Gazhonova VE, Efremova MP, Bachurina EM et al (2015) The possibilities of assessing the glandular type of the breast structure by sonotomography from the standpoint of the risk factor for breast cancer development. Ann Roentgenol Radiol 5:23–29 (article in Russian)
47. Golatta M, Baggs C, Schweitzer-Martin M et al (2015) Evaluation of an automated breast 3D-ultrasound system by comparing it with hand-held ultrasound (HHUS) and mammography. Arch Gynecol Obstet 291:889–895
48. Corsetti J, Ferrari A, Ghirardi M et al (2008) Role of ultrasonography in detecting mammographically occult breast carcinoma in women with dense breasts. Eur J Cancer 44:539–544
49. Gazhonova V, Efremova M, Hlustina E et al (2015) Automated Breast Volume Sonography (ABVS) – a new method of cancer diagnostics. Medical Visualization 2:67–77
50. Arps DP, Healy P, Zhao L et al (2013) Invasive ductal carcinoma with lobular features: a comparison study to invasive ductal and invasive lobular carcinomas of the breast. Breast Cancer Res Treat 138(3):719–726
51. Li CI, Anderson BO, Daling JR et al (2003) Trends in incidence rates of invasive lobular and ductal breast carcinoma. JAMA 289(11):1421–1424
52. Albayrak ZK, Onay HK, Karatag GY et al (2011) Invasive lobular carcinoma of the breast: mammographic and sonographic evaluation. Diagn Interv Radiol 17:232–238
53. Sickles EA (1986) Breast calcifications: mammographic evaluation. Radiology 160:289–293
54. Heywang-Koebrunner SH, Dershaw DD, Schreer I (2001) Microcalcification. In: Diagnostic breast imaging. Georg Thieme Verlag, New York, pp 434–452
55. Kheirelseid EH, Boggs JM, Curran C et al (2011) Younger age as a prognostic indicator in breast cancer: a cohort study. BMC Cancer 11:383–389
56. Lehman CD, Lee CI, Loving VA et al (2012) Accuracy and value of breast ultrasound for primary imaging evaluation of symptomatic women 30–39 years of age. AJR Am J Roentgenol 199:1169–1177
57. Kelemen LE, Pankratz VS, Sellers TA (2008) Age-specific trends in mammographic density: the Minnesota breast cancer family study. Am J Epidemiol 167:1027–1036
58. Stomper PC, D'Souza DJ, Di Nitto PA et al (1996) Analysis of parenchymal density on mammograms in 1353 women 25–79 years old. AJR Am J Roentgenol 167:1261–1265
59. Biglia N, Maggiorotto F, Liberale V et al (2013) Clinical-pathologic features, long term-outcome and surgical treatment in a large series of patients with invasive lobular carcinoma (ILC) and invasive ductal carcinoma (IDC). Eur J Surg Oncol 39(5):455–460
60. Selinko VL, Middleton LP, Dempsey PJ (2004) Role of sonography in diagnosing and staging invasive lobular carcinoma. J Clin Ultrasound 32(7):323–332
61. Fu L, Tsuchiya S, Matsuyama I et al (1998) Clinicopathological features and incidence of invasive lobular carcinoma in Japanese women. Pathol Int 48:348–354
62. Fu KL, Fu YS, Bassett LW et al (2005) Invasive malignancies. In: Bassett LW, Jackson VP, Fu SK

(eds) Diagnosis of the diseases of the breast, 2nd edn. Saunders, Philadelphia, pp 499–500

63. Weinstein SP, Orel SG, Heller R et al (2001) MR imaging of the breast in patients with invasive lobular carcinoma. AJR Am J Roentgenol 176: 399–406

64. Kumar V, Cotran RS, Robbins SL (1997) In: Kumar V, Cotran RS, Robbins SL (eds) Basic pathology, 6th edn. Philadelphia: Saunders, p 633

65. Butler RS, Venta LA, Wiley EL et al (1999) Sonographic evaluation of infiltrating lobular carcinoma. AJR Am J Roentgenol 172:325–330

66. Sickles EA (1991) The subtle and atypical mammographic features of invasive lobular carcinoma. Radiology 178:25–26

67. Watson L (2001) Breast cancer: diagnosis, treatment and prognosis. Radiol Technol 73:45–61

68. Paramagul CP, Helvie MA, Adler DD (1995) Invasive lobular carcinoma: sonographic appearance and role of sonography in improving diagnostic sensitivity. Radiology 195:231–234

69. Cho KR, Seo BK, Lee JY et al (2005) A comparative study of 2D and 3D ultrasonography for evaluation of solid breast masses. Eur J Radiol 54:365–370

70. Chapellier C, Balu-Maestro C, Bleuse A et al (2000) Ultrasonography of invasive lobular carcinoma of the breast: sonographic patterns and diagnostic value: report of 102 cases. Clin Imaging 24: 333–336

71. Krecke KN, Gisvold JJ (1993) Invasive lobular carcinoma of the breast: mammographic findings and extent of disease at diagnosis in 184 patients. AJR Am J Roentgenol 161:957–960

72. Chang JM, Moon WK, Cho N et al (2011) Breast cancers initially detected by hand-held ultrasound: detection performance of radiologists using automated breast ultrasound data. Acta Radiol 52: 8–14

73. Hersh MR (2004) Imaging the dense breast. Appl Radiol 33:22

74. Corsetti V, Ferrari A, Ghirardi M et al (2006) Role of ultrasonography in detecting mammographically occult breast carcinoma in women with dense breasts. Radiol Med 13(3):440–448

75. Zhang L, Liu YJ, Jiang SQ et al (2014) Ultrasound utility for predicting biological behavior of invasive ductal breast cancers. Asian Pacific J Cencer Prev 15(19):8057–8062

76. Tinnemans JG, Wobbes T, van der Sluis RF et al (1986) Multicentricity in nonpalpable breast carcinoma and its implications for treatment. Am J Surg 151:334–338

77. Dawson PJ, Baekey PA, Clark RA (1995) Mechanisms of multifocal breast cancer: an immunocytochemical study. Hum Pathol 26:965–969

78. Menezes GL, Van den Bosch MA, Postma EL et al (2013) Invasive ductolobular carcinoma of the breast: spectrum of mammographic, ultrasound and magnetic resonance imaging findings correlated with proportion of the lobular component. SpringerPlus 2:621. doi:10.1186/2193-1801-2-621

79. Robinson E, Rennert G, Rennert HS et al (1993) Survival of first and second primary breast cancer. Cancer 71:172–176

80. Peters NH, van Esser S, van den Bosch MA et al (2011) Preoperative MRI and surgical management in patients with nonpalpable breast cancer: the MO. Eur J Cancer 47(6):879–886

81. Isobe S, Tozaki M, Yamaguchi M et al (2011) Detectability of breast lesions under the nipple using an automated breast volume scanner: comparison with handheld ultrasonography. Jpn J Radiol 13(5):361–365. doi:10.1007/s11604-010-0555-5

82. Tozaki M, Fukuma E (2010) Accuracy of determining preoperative cancer extent measured by automated breast ultrasonography. Jpn J Radiol 13(10):771–773. doi:10.1007/s11604-010-0499-9

83. Glass AR (1994) Gynecomastia. Endocrinol Metab Clin North Am 23:825–837

84. Nuttall FQ (1979) Gynecomastia as a physical finding in normal men. J Clin Endocrinol Metab 48:338–340

85. Sørensen HT, Friis S, Olsen JH et al (1998) Risk of breast cancer in men with liver cirrhosis. Am J Gastroenterol 93:231–233

86. Andersen JA, Gram JB (1982) Male breast at autopsy. Acta Path Mictobiol Immunol Scand 90: 191–197

87. Albaum AH, Evans GF, Levy KR et al (1999) Mammographic appearances of male breast disease. Radiographics 19(3):559–568

88. Chen L, Chantra PK, Larsen LH et al (2006) Imaging characteristics of malignant lesions of the male breast. Radiographics 26(4):993–1006

89. Shaw A, Smith B, Howlett D (2011) Male breast carcinoma and the use of MRI. Radiol Case Rep 6:455–458

90. Nguyen C, Kettler MD, Swirsky ME et al (2013) Male breast disease. Pictorial review with radiologic-pathologic correlation. Radiographics 33:763–779

91. Lattin GE, Jesinger RA, Mattu R et al (2013) Diseases of the male breast: radiologic-pathologic correlation. Radiographics 33:461–489

92. Bembo SA, Carlson HE (2004) Gynaecomastia: its features and when and how to treat it. Cleve Clin J Med 71:511–517

93. Johnson RE, Murad MH (2009) Gynecomastia: pathophysiology, evaluation and management. Mayo Clin Proc 84:1010–1015

94. Braunstein GD (2007) Clinical practice: gynecomastia. N Engl J Med 357(12):1229–1230

95. Fentiman IS, Fourquet A, Hortobagyi GN (2006) Male breast cancer. Lancet 367:595–604

96. Giordano SH (2005) A review of the diagnosis and management of male breast cancer. Oncologist 10(7):471–479

97. Wershaw D, Berger P, Weutch B et al (1993) Mammographic finding in men with breast cancer. Am J Roentgenol 160:267–270

98. Welch ST, Babcock DS, Ballard ET (2004) Sonography of pediatric male breast masses: gynaecomastia and beyond. Pediatr Radiol 34:952–957

99. Foxman B, D'Arcy H, Gillespie B et al (2002) Lactation mastitis: occurrence and medical management among 946 breastfeeding women in the United States. Am J Epidemiol 155:103–114

100. Kinlay JR, O'Connell DL, Kinlay S (1998) Incidence of mastitis in breastfeeding women during the six months after delivery: a prospective cohort study. Med J Aust 169:310–312

101. Lawrence RA (1990) The puerperium, breastfeeding, and breast milk. Curr Opin Obstet Gynecol 2:23–30

102. Inch S, Renfrew MJ (1989) Common breastfeeding problems. In: Chalmers I, Enkin M, Keirse M (eds) Effective care in pregnancy and childbirth. Oxford University Press, Oxford, UK, pp 1375–1389

103. Trop I, Dugas A, David J et al (2011) Breast abscesses: evidence-based algorithms for diagnosis, management and follow-up. Radiographics 1: 1683–1699

104. Frank S, Mahdi R, Sherko K (2010) Imaging in patients with breast implants—results of the First International Breast (Implant) Conference 2009. Insights Imaging 1:93–97

105. Fisenko EP, Startseva OI (21012) Ultrasound of gel breast implants and soft tissues, 1st edn. "Firma Strom" JSC, Moscow 128 p

106. Stevens WG, Pacella SJ, Gear AJL et al (2008) Clinical experience with a fourth-generation textured silicone gel breast implant: a review of 1012 mentor memorygel breast implants. Aesthetic Surg J28:642–647

107. Sardanelli F, Boetes C, Borisch B et al (2010) Magnetic resonance imaging of the breast: recommendations from the EUSOMA working group. Eur J Cancer 46(8):1296–1316

108. Handel N (2007) The effect of silicone implants on the diagnosis, prognosis and treatment of breast cancer. Plast Reconstr Surg 120(Suppl1):81S–93S

109. Herborn CU, Marince KB, Erfmann D et al (2002) Breast augmentation and reconstructive surgery: MR imaging of implant rupture and malignancy. Eur Radiol 12:2198–2206

110. Yang N, Muradali D (2011) The augmented breast: a pictorial review of the abnormal and unusual. AJR Am J Roentgenol 196(4):451–460

111. Benedetto GD, Sara C, Luca G et al (2008) Comparative study of breast implant rupture using mammography, sonography, and magnetic resonance imaging: correlation with surgical findings. Breast J 14:532–537

112. Juanpere S, Perez E, Huc O (2011) Imaging of breast implants—a pictorial review. Insights Imaging 2:653–670. doi:10.1007/s13244-011-0122-3

113. Glynn C, Litherland J (2008) Imaging breast augmentation and reconstruction. Br J Radiol 81:587–595

114. Marini C, Cilotti A, Iacconi C et al (2006) Ultrasonographic appearance of breast implant complications. Ann Plast Surg 56:243–247

115. Singh-Ranger G, Mokbel K (2004) Capsular contraction following immediate reconstructive surgery for breast cancer – an association with methylene blue dye. Int Semin Surg Oncol 11;1(1):3 (An abstract)

116. Shiffman M (2009) Capsular contracture following augmnetation mannoplasty: etiology and pathogenesis. In: Breast augmentation: principles and practice. Springer. ISBN: 978-3-540-789482, pp 525–541

117. Spear SL, Baker JL Jr (1995) Classification of capsular contracture after prosthetic breast reconstruction. Plast Reconstr Surg 96(5):1119–1123

118. Gorczyca DP, Gorczyca SM, Gorczyca K (2007) The diagnosis of silicone breast implant rupture. Plast Reconstr Surg 120(Suppl1):49S–61S

119. Kubota K (2015) Diagnostic imaging of postoperative breast cancer with multiple modalities: recurrence, complications and normal postoperative appearances. ECR 2015, digital poster, C-0409. doi:10.1594/ecr2015/C-0409. doi-Link:http://dx.doi.org/10.1594/ecr2015/C-0409

120. Halyard MY, Bruce G, Harris Eleanor ER (2013) Local-Regional Recurrence (LRR) and Salvage Surgery—Breast Cancer. Expert Panel on Radiation Oncology–Breast: American College of Radiology ACR Appropriateness Criteria

121. Moran MS, Haffty BG (2002) Local-regional breast cancer recurrence: prognostic groups based on patterns of failure. Breast J8(2):81–87

122. van Tienhoven G, Voogd AC, Peterse JL et al (1999) Prognosis after treatment for loco-regional recurrence after mastectomy or breast conserving therapy in two randomised trials (EORTC 10801 and DBCG-82TM). EORTC Breast Cancer Cooperative Group and the Danish Breast Cancer Cooperative Group. Eur J Cancer 35(1):32–38

123. Brown MA, Ojeda-Fournier H, Dragana D (2014) Postsurgical breast and implant imaging. Published Online: 1 Mar 2014. doi:10.1002/9781118482858. ch11

124. Franque T, De Miguel C, Corzolluela R et al (1993) Spiculated lesions of the breast: mammographic-pathologic correlation. Radiograhics 13:841–852

125. Cha ES, Kang BJ, Kim HS et al (2007) Contrast enhanced MRI findings of radial scar: correlation with histopathology. Biomed Imaging Interv J 3: S12–S402

ABVS technology has some limitations. Automated breast ultrasound is limited in women with macromastia and pronounced ptosis [1, 2]. Isobe et al. [3] pointed out some difficulties in the scanning of large breasts and the retroareolar area despite the large scanning surface. Furthermore, they presume that even with optimal scanning technique, the peripheral areas of the breast parenchyma are not fully covered by ABVS [3]. Therefore, some areas of the breast, such as deep lateral areas, do not have proper visualization and complete coverage using ABVS. The scanning field of 17 cm does not allow the inclusion of the entire volume of the breast in a single scan for patients with a bra cup size (F) or more (Fig. 5.1). This reduces the diagnostic value of ABVS when compared with conventional two-dimensional ultrasound [3]. In our view this arises only with coronal scans, in which the outer portions of the gland are not so compressed and could not be evaluated so thoroughly, but we used some special projections in which a patient lies on her side for scanning the lateral portion of the gland or shifting the breast laterally for scanning medial portions of the gland. Similarly we use the technique of shifting the breast down for scanning the upper part and upward for scanning the inferior part. If a mass is detected in the lower or inner quadrants on the mammogram, it is possible to supplement the study by scanning from the mediolateral view or separately capture the lower quadrants. These scanning principles will result

in better visualization of the tissues of the subsequent zones [4]. Therefore, we recommend in such cases to follow the principle of sequential study of all zones of interest with maximum capture of all areas and obtaining additional views of quadrants not included in the initial view.

There is no experience in examining the axillary region with ABVS, although it is of special importance in breast cancer diagnosis. Today, sentinel node biopsy is the standard therapy for women at the preoperative stage with a negative nodal status, which requires ultrasound of the axilla [5]. Furthermore, lymph node alterations may be the first sign in mammographically and/or sonographically occult breast cancer or other malignant diseases. Therefore, additional conventional ultrasound of the axilla would be necessary after a suspicious ABVS scan. This drawback of ABVS is noted by all researchers, and this limits the possibility of using this method for screening [6–14].

In our clinical experience, we faced a case of false-negative diagnosis of multifocal breast cancer localized in the axillary process. Retrospective analysis of the whole array of stored ultrasound data showed that the tumor was located outside the scanning field. It was impossible to cover the axillary process completely at a volume scan, and therefore we could not view the tumor by processing the entire array of 3D data (Fig. 5.2). To avoid such false-negative cases, the patient should initially be examined with conventional

© Springer International Publishing Switzerland 2017
V. Gazhonova, *3D Automated Breast Volume Sonography*, DOI 10.1007/978-3-319-41971-8_5

2D ultrasound followed by an ABVS study with additional scanning of the breast's axillary process, which may reveal multifocal tumor growth in the patient.

Additionally, shadowing artifacts occur in the retroareolar region despite the special algorithm (adaptive nipple shadow reduction tool) used for reduction of nipple shadowing and to a certain extent in the remaining breast volume. Therefore, a certain proportion of breast parenchyma may be lost in the volume data. This may reduce the diagnostic potential in comparison to handheld ultrasound. As previously mentioned, a special technique for acquiring volumetric data was suggested. Maximum lateralization of the nipple is used to avoid these artifacts and reduces no-show zones (Fig. 5.3).

During an automatic scan, movement or conversation artifacts arise in some cases, which adversely affect the perception of 3D data (Figs. 5.4 and 5.5). The lack of contact of the scanning membrane with the skin of the gland can cause some artifacts in the so-called "dumb" zone, such as in scar deformity of the breast after lumpectomy or sectoral resection, in severe retraction of the nipple and breast deformation in infiltrating breast cancer, in breast implants, in expanders, and sometimes in cases of severe pain in mastitis (Fig. 5.6). In these cases, you should conduct an examination using the standard 2D technique.

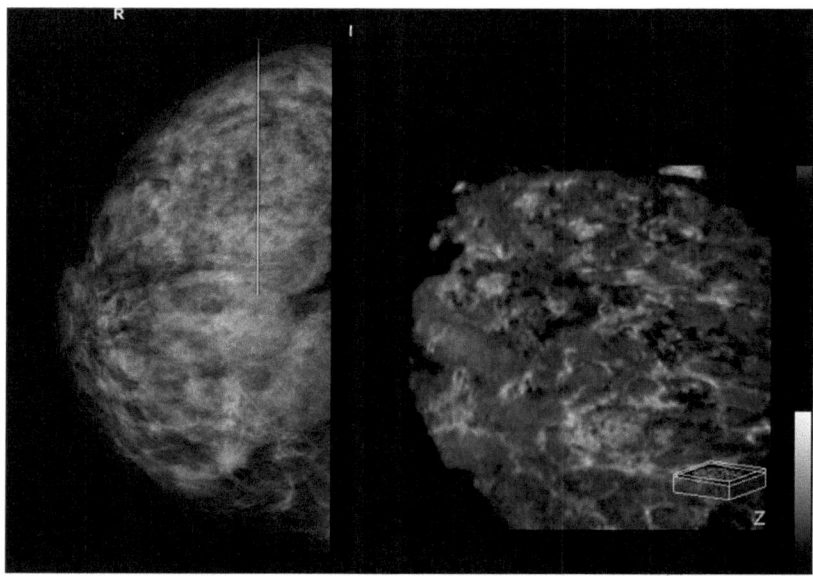

Fig. 5.1 Side-by-side comparison of the X-ray mammography craniocaudal direct view and R SUP (superior-to-inferior view) ABVS images of the right breast in a patient with macromastia. The ABVS transducer covers only half of the field covered by MMG

Fig. 5.2 Multifocal IDC (3T1N0M0, Luminal B, G2) with localization in the axillaris process that was missed on ABVS due to the peripheral location. Comparison of HHUS, ABVS, and MMG. (**a**) Multiple hypoechoic tumors with indistinct margins with a hyperechoic halo sign and increased anteroposterior diameter. (**b**) Sonoelastography of the lesions. Increased stiffness of both tumors, colored deep blue. (**c**) Bilateral ABVS in coronal anteroposterior projection. A symmetrical distribution of the breast parenchyma, absence of additional lesions, and retraction phenomenon. (**d, e**) Side-by-side comparison of mammographic and ABVS images in the corresponding projections. (**d**) Direct CC MMG (*lower part*) and R SUP ABVS (*upper part*). (**e**) MLo MMG (*right part*) and LMO ABVS (*left part*)

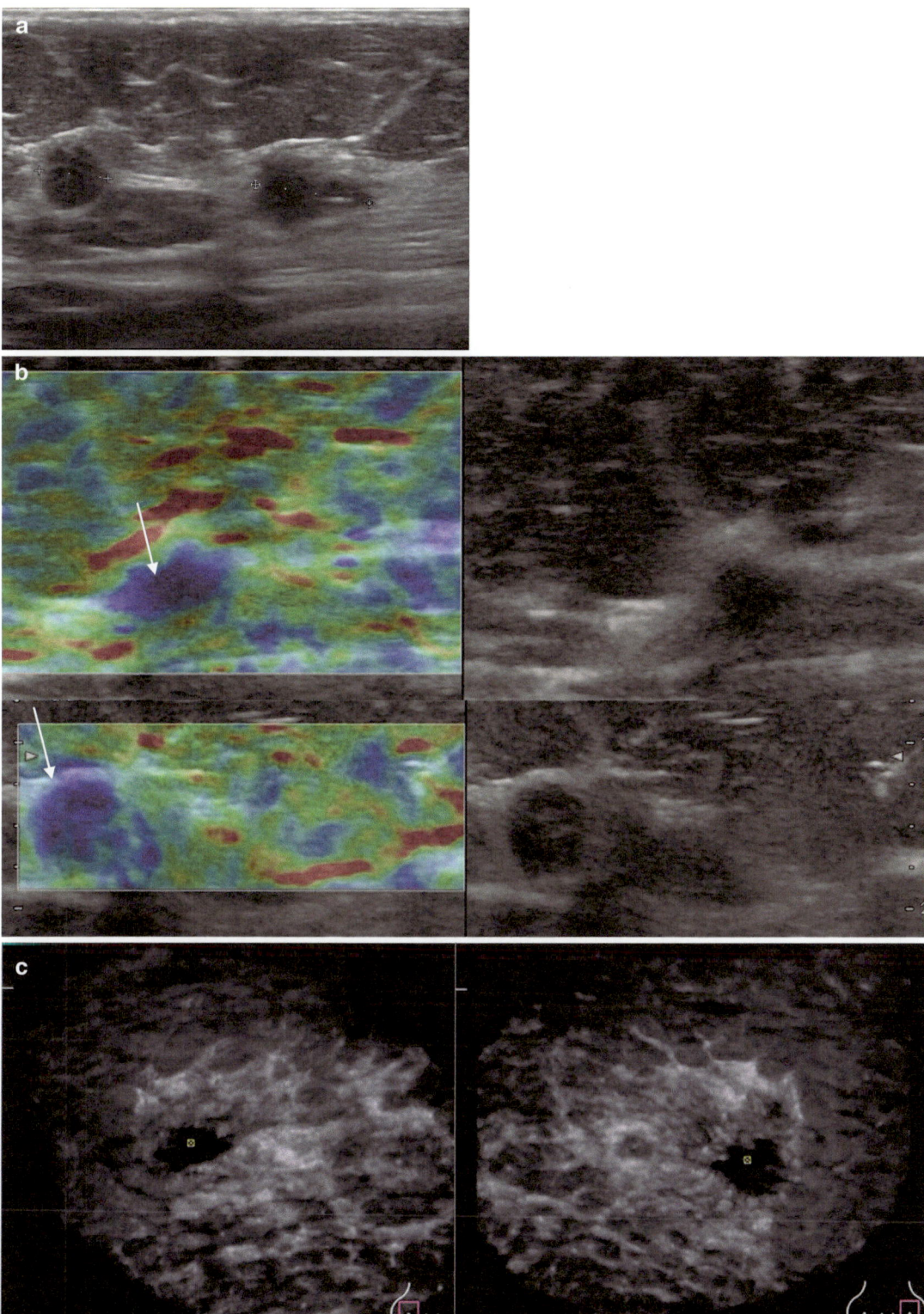

Fig. 5.2 (continued)

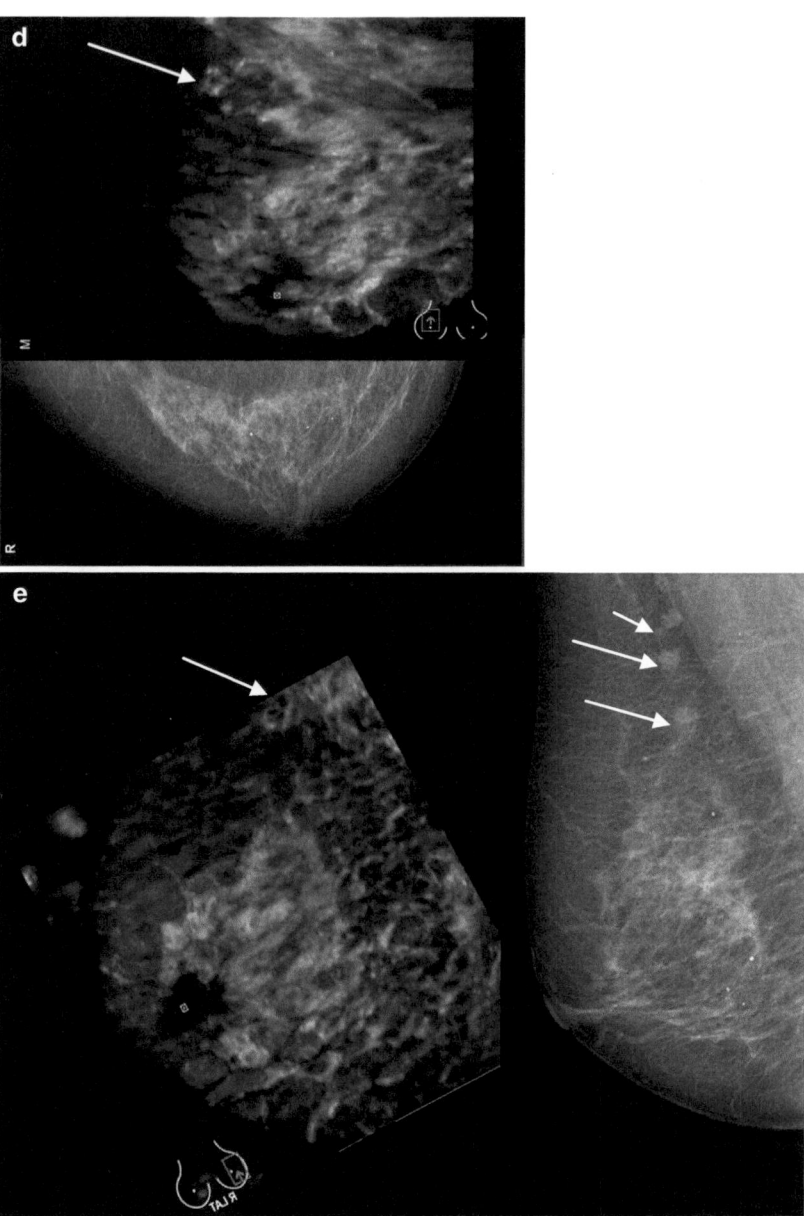

The ABVS technique, despite its high sensitivity, has low specificity with a high number of false-positive findings. A large number of time-consuming second-look ultrasound examinations have to be taken into account. The lack of standardized interpretation criteria and technical artifacts in the volume data set lead to low specificity of 52.8 % [14]. In all studies the proportion of cases to controls was not the representative of the whole population. Therefore, the results concerning the sensitivity, specificity, and rate of second-look ultrasounds cannot be applied to the general population and hence must be carefully interpreted. This problem may be solved through second readings by an independent examiner. To reduce the number of false-positive findings, we recommend using the full range of diagnostic ultrasound possibilities included in the US device in one study. Some studies include only ABVS in the examination protocol without HHUS data.

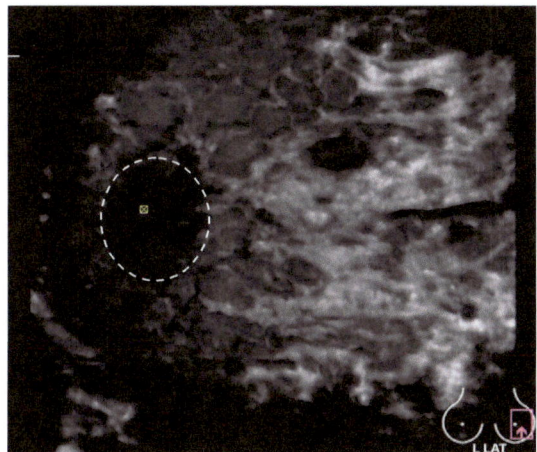

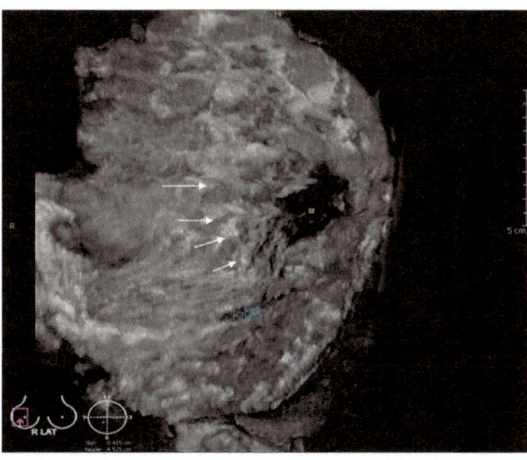

Fig. 5.3 An example of a nipple shadow artifact. A large anechoic zone is seen around the nipple in the L Lat scan (left latero-medial oblique) scan. Note the nipple is not properly lateralized; this results in the large "no-show" zone

Fig. 5.5 An example of artifacts from a phone conversation during the study. Small waves disturb the picture of the breast parenchyma

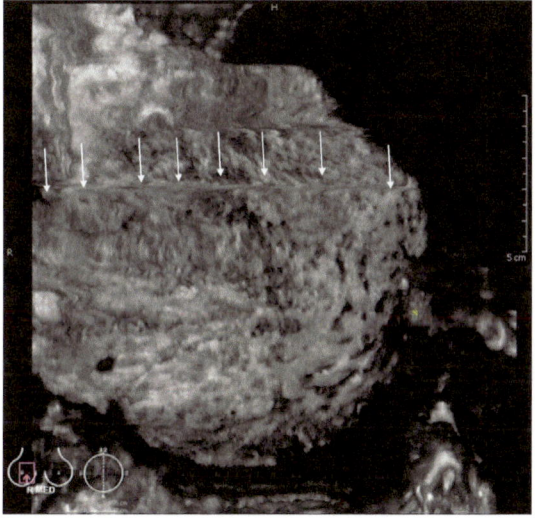

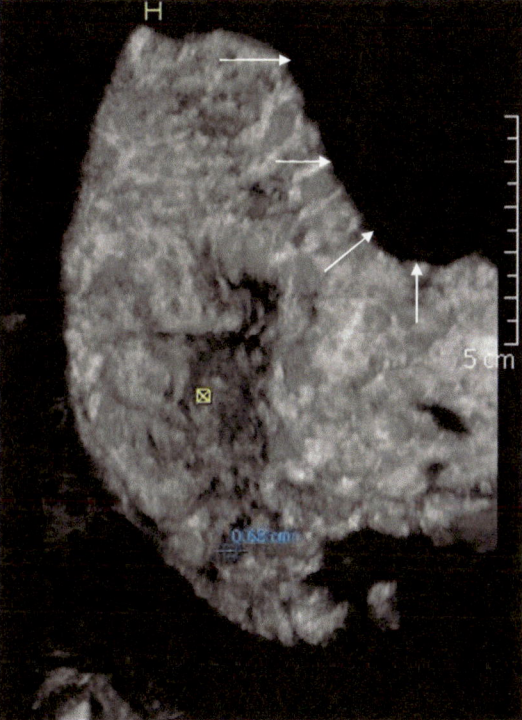

Fig. 5.4 An example of an artifact from a movement during acquisition of the 3D data. A large strip line is seen in the upper portion of the left breast obtained in the latero-medial position (*white arrow*). Small waves are also seen above that line; these also result from speaking during the acquisition (*arrowheads*)

Fig. 5.6 An example of "dumb" zone artifacts due to the lack of contact of the scanning membrane with the skin of the breast. Note the large region in the upper part of the small breast (A cup size) after acquisition of the latero-medial oblique view

And with that the ability to immediately further explore a questionable lesion by modifying factors such as the compression, the orientation of the probe, and the machine's setting while acquiring the image in real-time Doppler imaging or sonoelastography is lost [14].

As we have already mentioned, 2D ultrasound is the first step with additional options for analysis of the blood supply to the tumor and its density assessment, and ABVS is the second step to detect microcalcifications and "retraction" phenomenon. This, in turn, somewhat increases the length of the study of the breasts but also increases the specificity of the ultrasound examination [4, 15]. In terms of the future broad clinical application of the ABVS technique for the diagnosis of breast cancer, the relatively small number of false-negative cases, evidenced by numerous studies, is encouraging [16–22].

Despite the well-known advantages, ABVS is a time-consuming technique, just like conventional two-dimensional ultrasound. This technique requires the training of not only medical but also nursing staff to reduce the technical load of the procedures on the physician. A number of works on ABVS pointed out that 3D ABVS takes less time than conventional 2D ultrasound [7, 14]. But no full answers were found concerning examination and interpretation time. While exploring these techniques, the time for acquisition and for analysis was significantly reduced when we gained experience, but still the time of the study was not less than 30 min. Clinical experience shows that more time is consumed by analysis and comparison with X-ray mammogram data. We observed a direct correlation of increased study time with a larger breast size, changes on the X-ray mammogram, and suspected malignancy. If multiple lesions are present in the breast, the time of the study was prolonged.

With the 3D US technique, questions of storage of digital information arise. The mean volume of a single study is an average of about 2 GB. Unlike digital breast tomosynthesis, one has to maintain tomographic information of six standard views, and this requires a more optimal technical solution. In this regard it is not clear at

the moment how the digital archives of ABVS tomograms, mammograms, and digital breast tomosynthesis will be matched. In addition, the widespread use of this technique is still limited by the small number of ultrasonic devices with the function of automatic volume scanning.

All the abovementioned factors mean that at the moment ABVS must be regarded as an experimental approach. ABVS is far from being accepted in medical practice, and its application still lacks solid data from comprehensive studies.

In order to move this technique forward, there is a definite need for further research, prospective studies recruiting larger patient's cohorts, and a multicenter design with multi-observer analysis.

Bibliography

1. Wöhrle NK, Hellerhoff K, Notohamiprodjo M et al (2010) Automated breast volume scanner (ABVS): a new approach for breast imaging. Radiologe 50:973–981
2. Chang JM, Moon WK, Cho N et al (2011) Breast cancers initially detected by hand-held ultrasound: detection performance of radiologists using automated breast ultrasound data. Acta Radiol 52:8–14
3. Isobe S, Tozaki M, Yamaguchi M et al (2011) Detectability of breast lesions under the nipple using an automated breast volume scanner: comparison with handheld ultrasonography. Jpn J Radiol 13(5):361–365
4. Gazhonova VE, Bachurina EM, Hlustina EM et al (2014) Automatic sonotomography of the breast (3D ABVS). Part 1. Integration of US method in the radiological imaging standards. Polyclinic Special issue 3, "X-ray diagnostics", pp 42–48 (article in Russian)
5. Wang ZL, Xw JH, Li JL et al (2012) Comparison of automated breast volume scanning to hand-held ultrasound and mammography. Radiol Med 13(8):1287–1293. doi:10.1007/s11547-012-0836-4
6. Maturo VG, Zusmer NR, Gilson AJ et al (1980) Ultrasound of the whole breast utilizing a dedicated automated breast scanner. Radiology 137:457–463
7. Tozaki M, Isobe S, Yamaguchi M et al (2010) Optimal scanning technique to cover the whole breast using an automated breast volume scanner. Jpn J Radiol 28:325–328. Deutsche GesellschaftfürUltraschall in der Medizin (DEGUM) MehrstufenkonzeptMammasonographie
8. Wojcinski S, Farrokh A, Hille U et al (2011) The automated breast volume scanner (ABVS): initialexperie ncesinlesiondetectioncomparedwithconventionalhand heldB-modeultrasound: a pilot study of 50 cases. Int J Wom Health 13:337–346

9. Shin HJ, Kim HH, Cha JH et al (2011) Automated ultrasound of the breast for diagnosis: interobserver agreement on lesion detection and characterization. AJR Am J Roentgenol 13(3):747–754. doi:10.2214/AJR.10.5841

10. Golatta M, Franz D, Harcos A et al (2013) Interobserver reliability of automated breast volume scanner (ABVS) interpretation and agreement of ABVS findings with hand held breast ultrasound (HHUS), mammography and pathology results. Eur J Radiol 13(8):332–336

11. Lin X, Wang J, Han F et al (2012) Analysis of eighty-one cases with breast lesions using automated breast volume scanner and comparison with handheld ultrasound. Eur J Radiol 13(5):873–878. doi:10.1016/j.ejrad.2011.02.038

12. Wang HY, Jiang YX, Zhu QL et al (2012) Differentiation of benign and malignant breast lesions: a comparison between automatically generated breast volume scans and hand held ultrasound examinations. Eur J Radiol 13(11):3190–3200. doi:10.1016/j.ejrad.2012.01.034

13. Lin X, Wang J, Han F et al (2012) Analysis of eighty-one cases with breast lesions using automated breast volume scanner and comparison with handheld ultrasound. Eur J Radiol 13(5):873–878

14. Wojcinski S, Gyapong S, Farrokh A et al (2013) Diagnostic performance and inter-observer concordance in lesion detection with the automated breast volume scanner (ABVS). BMC Med Imaging 13:36

15. Gazhonova V, Efremova M, Hlustina E et al (2015) Automated Breast Volume Sonography (ABVS) – a new method of cancer diagnostics. Medical Visualization 2:67–77 (article in Russian)

16. Jacobs OE, Rozhkova NI, Maso ML et al (2014) The experience of virtual sonography of the breast use. Ann Roentgenol Radiol 1:23–32 (article in Russian)

17. Jacobs OE, Kaprin AD, Rozhkova NI et al (2014) Virtual sonography of the breast. The experience of clinical use. Medical Visualization 2: 22–31 (article in Russian)

18. Jackson VP, Kelly-Fry E, Rothschild PA et al (1986) Automated breast sonography using a 7.5-MHz PVDF transducer: preliminary clinical evaluation. Work in progress. Radiology 159:679–684

19. Chou YH, Tiu CM, Chen J et al (2007) Automated full-field breast ultrasonography: the past and the present. J Med Ultrasound 15:31–44

20. Shin HJ, Kim HH, Cha JH (2015) Current status of automated breast ultrasonography. Ultrasonography 34(3):165–172

21. Kelly KM, Dean J, Comulada WS et al (2010) Breast cancer detection using automated whole breast ultrasound and mammography in radiographically dense breasts. Eur Radiol 20:734–742

22. Kaplan SS (2014) Automated whole breast ultrasound. Radiol Clin North Am 52:539–546

Conclusion

6

ABVS is a feasible method that may in the future be integrated into the workflow of a breast cancer center. ABVS guarantees high patient safety as there is no exposure to ionizing radiation and no injection of a contrast medium. ABVS is a highly sensitive method for breast cancer detection by both the "retraction" phenomenon and visualization of structural impairments in the whole breast. Women with dense breast tissue may benefit from ABVS because of improved workflow efficiency and lack of operator dependence. We proposed the use of ABVS with X-ray MMG together in order to increase the sensitivity and specificity of breast cancer detection.

ABVS is advantageous compared with HHUS in that it is less dependent on the examiners and it has excellent reproducibility. A good interobserver agreement is established for ABVS. A special wide aperture high-frequency probe produces sufficient image quality and resolution, and with its help the location of lesions can be determined more accurately by obtaining images of the overall breast. Patients with malignant breast tumors larger than 5 cm who undergo neoadjuvant chemotherapy may benefit from the automated technique because the handheld device has a smaller footprint (5 cm) and therefore is limited in the evaluation of the extent of disease. Patients with multiple masses might benefit from faster examination times than those of handheld ultrasound. With the ABVS technique, the topography of surgical planning can be made easier.

ABVS may make ultrasound available to a larger number of women. Image acquisition with ABVS can be efficiently performed by a medical assistant. The performance of second readings by additional examiners and follow-up evaluations are unproblematic, which is important in screening programs. Moreover, ABVS allows a delayed interpretation of the images at any time.

ABVS coronal slices may assist in precise biopsy or when planning surgery.

Many researchers believe that the ultrasound breast tomosynthesis technique, or ABVS, can already today be integrated in the practice of outpatient oncology centers and multidisciplinary hospitals. Unfortunately the role of ABVS in breast cancer diagnosis screening programs has not yet been determined. In order to move this technique forward, there is a definite need for further research, prospective studies recruiting larger patients' cohorts, and a multicenter design with multi-observer analysis.

One can easily imagine that in the future, possibly after further improvement, this technique will be used for screening younger patients under 40 years old and women with dense breasts, and additional studies such as CT and MRI mammography will be reserved only for cases with inconclusive ultrasound data.

© Springer International Publishing Switzerland 2017
V. Gazhonova, *3D Automated Breast Volume Sonography*, DOI 10.1007/978-3-319-41971-8_6

Index